100 Questions & Answers About Brain Tumors

Virginia Stark-Vance, MD
M.L. Dubay

JONES AND BARTLETT PUBLISHERS
Sudbury, Massachusetts
BOSTON   TORONTO   LONDON   SINGAPORE

World Headquarters
Jones and Bartlett
Publishers
40 Tall Pine Drive
Sudbury, MA 01776
info@jbpub.com
www.jbpub.com

Jones and Bartlett
Publishers Canada
2406 Nikanna Road
Mississauga, ON L5C 2W6
CANADA

Jones and Bartlett
Publishers International
Barb House, Barb Mews
London W6 7PA
UK

Library of Congress Cataloging-in-Publication Data
Stark-Vance, Virginia.
   100 questions & answers about brain tumors / Virginia Stark-Vance,
M.L. Dubay.
      p. cm.
Includes bibliographical references and index.
   ISBN 0-7637-2308-8
   1. Brain—Tumors—Popular works. I. Title: One hundred questions and
answers about brain tumors. II. Dubay, M.L. (Mary Louise) III. Title.
   RC280.B7S79 2003
   616.99'481—dc21

                                                          2003008137

The authors, editors, and publisher have made every effort to provide accurate information. However, they are not responsible for errors, omissions, or for any outcomes related to the use of the contents of this book and take no responsibility for the use of any products described herein. Treatments and side effects described in this book may not be applicable to all patients; likewise, some patients may require a dose or experience a side effect that is not described herein. The reader should confer with his or her own physician regarding specific treatments and side effects. Drugs and medical devices are discussed that may have limited availability or be controlled by the Food and Drug Administration (FDA) for use only in a research study or clinical trial. The drug information presented has been derived from reference sources, recently published data, and pharmaceutical research data. Research, clinical practice, and government regulations often change the accepted standard in this field. When consideration is being given to use any drug in the clinical setting, the healthcare provider or reader is responsible for determining FDA status of the drug, reading the package insert, reviewing prescribing information for the most up-to-date recommendations on dose, precautions, and contraindications, and determining the appropriate usage for the product. This is especially important in the case of drugs that are new or seldom used. Comments from a patient or patients other than the authors that may be used in this text are the opinions of the commenter and should not be construed as representative of the authors' or publisher's viewpoint.

Production Credits
Acquisitions Editor: Christopher Davis
Production Editor: Elizabeth Platt
Cover Design: Philip Regan
Manufacturing Buyer: Therese Bräuer
Composition: Northeast Compositors
Printing and Binding: Malloy Lithographing
Cover Printer: Malloy Lithographing

Printed in the United States of America
08 07 06 05 04   10 9 8 7 6 5 4 3 2 1

Contents

Questions 1–6 cover the background about brain tumors, including:

- What is a brain tumor?
- Can any part of the brain have a tumor? Where do most brain tumors occur in the brain? Are there areas of the brain that are more dangerous to have a tumor?
- What causes a brain tumor?

Questions 7–14 discuss how brain tumors are diagnosed and classified, including:

- What are the symptoms of brain tumors? Do all brain tumors cause headache?
- What is a neurological examination?
- What are the most common types of primary brain tumors?

Questions 15–22 explore the various techniques used to look at brain tumors, such as:

- Why do I need both a CT scan and an MRI scan?
- How often should I have a follow-up MRI scan?
- What is a PET scan, and should I have one? Why does my doctor use MRI scans and not PET scans to evaluate my tumor?

Questions 23–32 discuss what you can expect from brain surgery, including:

- What are the potential complications of a neurosurgical procedure?
- Are there some tumors that can be surgically cured? Is a tumor that cannot be resected always incurable?
- Why do I still need therapy if all the malignant cells were removed?

v

100 Questions & Answers About Brain Tumors uses a novel approach to transmit information to patients and their families who seek understanding about myriad topics—from day-to-day living with a brain tumor, to coping with treatment side effects, to talking to friends, to changing priorities, and everything else in between. A patient's comments and stories are interspersed with the doctor's explanations.

Patients, caregivers, families, and friends are guaranteed to learn from the answers and commentaries found here. Also, the healthcare team treating brain tumor patients will learn about those unasked questions that patients were afraid to ask, were too embarrassed to ask, or forgot to ask during their hospital stay or office visit.

During my fifteen years in the brain tumor community, I've witnessed an evolution in our society's acceptance of individuals diagnosed with a brain tumor. In the late 1980s, there was a reluctance to talk freely about it. A brain tumor was more than a disease—it was a stigma. A brain tumor can affect emotions, intellect, personality—the very essence of a person—and people are frightened if they witness such changes, especially if they don't understand the cause. Location and histology of the tumor are determinant factors in such changes; their onset may be gradual or sudden. However, because few people were talking about brain tumors, the general public knew little about them.

Compared to other cancers, brain tumors have a relatively low incidence, making it an "orphan disease" by government standards, which classify any disease with an annual incidence of less than 200,000 as an orphan disease. Our numbers today estimate 186,000 diagnoses of brain tumors annually, which includes over 120 different types of brain tumors.

I personally credit Mr. Lee Atwater for beginning to change society's attitude about brain tumors when he went public about his disease. In the early 1990s, Mr. Atwater was Chairman of the Republican National Committee under President George H. W. Bush. He was the first prominent person to announce that he was battling a brain tumor. I remember seeing him on the cover of *Life* magazine; I knew that his candor would make a difference for future patients. According to published accounts at the time, Mr. Atwater had a reputation for being a "bad boy" in politics, but I firmly believe he made amends for any misdeeds he may have done by coming forward and empowering people to speak openly about brain tumors.

My, how far we've come. The past decade has brought new diagnostic and microsurgical tools and techniques, more effective treatment therapies for some brain tumors, a proliferation of brain tumor-focused organizations and support groups, and many patient education publications, including a significant library of booklets and pamphlets written by the American Brain Tumor Association. And, most notably, having a brain tumor is no longer a stigma. Rather, this past decade has produced a generation of information-seekers who have a driving need to have their questions answered.

The intriguing aspect of this book is its approach: provocative questions and honest answers given by a clinician and a patient. This resource for brain tumor patients and their families brings home the fact that no one needs to feel that he or she is battling this disease alone.

Ms. Dubay has encountered the disease, the healthcare professionals, the medical system, and the unasked questions of family and friends. She answers questions and provides commentaries on issues that only a patient would know how to address. The brain tumor community-at-large will benefit from her first-hand knowledge.

Dr. Stark-Vance responds to questions with clarity, candor, and sound medical expertise. She does not sugarcoat her answers, nor does she underestimate a patient's need to know. This resource is a valuable new tool in the patients' battle against brain tumors—helpful, supportive, and honest.

This book is a must-have reference for those living in the brain tumor community.

Naomi Berkowitz
Executive Director
American Brain Tumor Association
March 2003

"You have a brain tumor." How chilling those words are the first time you hear them!

If you are like many patients, your initial response is likely to be sheer terror. Most people have no idea what having a brain tumor really means. You may wonder whether you have just been handed a death sentence. After giving you the diagnosis, your doctor may keep on talking, but it will most likely be difficult for you to keep listening.

Soon enough, though, you'll want to know more. Over the years, I have taken care of a lot of people with cancer. In my experience, most of them want to be active participants in their treatment. Informed patients—people who understand what is happening in their bodies, what their treatments are designed to do, and what the future is likely to bring—often cope better and may even have better outcomes. Family members who know what to expect are better equipped to offer care and support.

100 Questions & Answers About Brain Tumors is the place to come for the information you need. The language is clear, and the science is rigorous. Dr. Virginia Stark-Vance offers examples from her own oncology practice as she explains how brain tumors form, what your treatment options are, why you should consider a clinical trial, and where the uncertainties and the controversies lie. Her co-author, M.L. Dubay, has had a brain tumor herself, and she describes her own experiences here, providing a glimpse of what the diagnosis means on a day-to-day basis. The stories are honest, moving, and sometimes very funny.

I had the privilege of meeting Dr. Stark-Vance when she was on the staff of the National Cancer Institute in the Washington, D.C. area. I was supervising the care of former Congressman Mike Synar. Mike was a close personal friend of mine, and he came to me when he first developed the blinding headaches that were eventually diagnosed as a rare and aggressive brain tumor. Virginia was his oncologist. I was moved not only by her professional competence, but by her compassion and dedication.

Mike was one of those patients who wanted to know everything about his tumor and the available treatments. He asked a lot of questions about what the future held, he tolerated his chemotherapy well, and we were able to control the nausea and pain that can sometimes be debilitating.

But we could not keep Mike alive. And that, in the most personal of ways, tells me that we must step up the pace of research into brain tumors and continue our medical advances. The yardstick by which we measure our success is clear: the extent to which we can eliminate tumors without damaging brain function.

Treatment for brain tumors dates back many millennia. The archeological record tells us that brain surgery was performed in the Neolithic period, 9,000 years ago, and that patients survived the intervention. Chemotherapy is, of course, much newer—barely 50 years ago, doctors used it for the first time, administering nitrogen mustard through the carotid artery.

We've come a long way since then, but the available drug treatments are still too toxic and not nearly effective enough. When I was commissioner of the Food and Drug Administration, we sometimes approved drugs for cancer that worked only about 15% of the time. That was better than nothing, we felt, but it certainly wasn't good enough.

Fortunately, the options for treating brain tumors are likely to keep getting better. The fruits of our investment in molecular biology are only beginning to pay off. We're identifying new targets where drugs may be effectively delivered, and we're making great progress in finding new ways to deliver them. Down the road, safer and more effective treatments will surely become available. For the first time, researchers are exploring the possibility of administering cancer drugs in doses that are large enough to be effective—and small enough not to be toxic.

I hope the day will come soon when we establish national laboratories dedicated to deciphering the biology and chemistry of cancer. Not all brain tumors are malignant, of course, but some so-called benign tumors can be deadly, so there are a lot of research needs to be met in this area, too. I'd also like to see the pharmaceutical industry move faster to develop and test promising new drugs.

But today, you need the best that medicine has to give you. And you need trustworthy information about your options presented in a way that you can understand. That is what you will find in this book. For that, Dr. Stark-Vance and M.L. Dubay deserve our thanks.

David Kessler, MD, JD
Dean, Yale Medical School
New Haven, Connecticut

When a colleague asks me to see someone newly diagnosed with a brain tumor, I meet someone whose life has been dramatically altered by this terrible diagnosis. Regardless of whether the patient is a flight attendant, software engineer, or hairdresser, he or she must absorb a vast quantity of information about the diagnosis and treatment options within a very short period of time. However, most patients are recovering from surgery and cannot be expected to remember the details of our discussion. Over the course of the next several days, I will introduce several concepts about brain tumor diagnosis and treatment options to the patient and family, and those discussions form the basis for this book.

Brain tumor patients have some disadvantages, compared with other patients with cancer. Although there are over 100 different types of brain tumors, there are only about 18,000 people diagnosed in the United States each year with a primary brain tumor—less than 2% of all cancer cases. Of course, it is fortunate that brain tumors *are* relatively rare, but they are disproportionately lethal, resulting in 13,000 deaths per year. Development of new drugs for the treatment of rare diseases is not a high priority for many pharmaceutical companies, and brain tumor researchers must compete for grants against researchers for other cancers that claim many more lives. Moreover, there are no effective screening tools for the early detection of brain tumors. There are no blood tests or tumor markers that may be included in an annual physical. Most significantly, the disability that results from a brain tumor can limit the access to treatment or even the ability to comprehend the diagnosis and treatment options.

Neurosurgeons have long recognized that their ability to remove the tumor for some patients may be limited. New imaging and surgical techniques have expanded the options for some patients, but the residual tumor cells that often spread through the surrounding normal brain require other forms of treatment. While all surgery has its risks, the possibility of damaging healthy brain is one of the most sobering aspects of brain tumor treatment.

Radiation therapy and chemotherapy also have significant limitations in the treatment of brain tumors. There is no question that, in many cases, such toxic treatments prolong survival, and the quality of life for many patients following treatment remains excellent. However, the number of patients who are cured of their disease is disappointingly small. It is unlikely that the current modalities of surgery, radiation therapy, and drug therapy can be modified in some novel arrangement to substantially increase the cure rate. Thus, new treatment strategies aimed at targeting the cancer cell more specifically may yield better tumor control and less toxicity.

Even with the less-than-optimal treatment strategies currently available, some patients will live long enough to take advantage of new discoveries. In 1993 temozolomide was a new drug showing promise in the treatment of malignant glioma in Europe. Only six years later temozolomide (Temodar) received approval for the treatment of recurrent anaplastic astrocytoma in the United States. Since then, Temodar has become a widely accepted chemotherapy drug in the treatment of malignant glioma. Another drug, Gliadel, a dissolvable chemotherapy wafer originally approved for surgical implantation for recurrent malignant glioma, recently received FDA approval for newly diagnosed malignant glioma. Its approval was based on the results of a clinical trial that showed an improvement in long-term survival. These are small steps, to be sure, but they nevertheless indicate that some progress is being made.

In this book, I wanted to explain and illustrate the concepts that brain tumor patients need to grasp to become active participants in their treatment plan. There are many more good questions that could have been included, and some of the answers given could be more detailed. However, there are excellent sources of information on the Internet that provide more in-depth discussion and I am quite happy to refer interested readers to the sources listed in the appendix. Also, I realize that questions I included, such as a question about deep vein thrombosis, represent *my* bias because I want patients to know about this common complication. Even with the help I received from my local medical librarian, Claire, I am fully responsible for any errors or omissions!

I am grateful for my co-author, M.L., who is smart, funny, gorgeous, well organized, and "just happens" to have a malignant brain tumor. M.L. reminds me so much of my sister Margaret that I had to keep reminding myself that I could not ask to borrow her clothes. She could be an articulate spokesperson for any worthy cause, but I'm thankful that she has become an advocate for brain tumor patients. Even with all her responsibilities at Nortel Networks, she somehow found the time to write this book. It's amazing to me that she could take on another project because she is very involved with her family, her church, and her community. If I were M.L.'s friend or sister, I would want to read a book like this just to find out everything I could about how to help her.

I have the privilege of working with an outstanding group of neurosurgeons, radiation oncologists, neurologists, and neuroradiologists in the Dallas-Fort Worth area who have dedicated themselves to improving the lives of brain tumor patients in our community. I am in awe of their talent and deeply in debt to those who have involved me in the care of their patients. Several of these colleagues provided questions and answers from their own experience with patients. Dr. Timothy Nichols, Dr. John Torrisi, Dr. Ed Gilbert, Dr. Warren Whitlow, Dr. Tom Moore, and Dr. Mike Desaloms offered suggestions for the radiation therapy, neuroradiology, and neurosurgery sections.

My daughter Joy, my sister Donna, and my brother-in-law Tom made helpful suggestions for the manuscript, and Tom wrote much of the glossary to help us meet our deadline. My son Ted provided me with 24/7 technical support to keep my iMac and DSL up and running. My office manager Paula took on much more responsibility so that I could free up more time to work on the book, and, as any solo practitioner knows, any success I achieve is because of this great lady. The editorial staff at Jones and Bartlett, Chris Davis and Elizabeth Platt, were extremely supportive in all aspects of the project—and allowed M.L. and me a lot more freedom that we expected.

To my patients at the National Cancer Institute, in Dallas, and in Fort Worth: thank you for allowing me to share in your life. I don't play golf or tennis, but I'm thrilled that you do. I don't have intricate tattoos, but I admire yours. I love to see your floppy hats, colorful scarves, and Texas-flag do-rags. I look forward to seeing which NASCAR driver is featured this week on your tee shirt. I love to hear about the Alaskan cruise, the trip to Vegas, and the scuba diving expedition. Thanks for sending the quilts, the flowers, and the coffee mugs. Thanks for sharing pineapple pie, homemade tamales, and deer jerky. Thanks for sending birth announcements, graduation announcements, wedding invitations, and Christmas cards for the last nine years. Most of all, thank you for showing me, every day, why it is so important to find a cure for brain tumors.

Also, I would like to express my deep gratitude to the family and friends of Mike Synar, the U.S. Congressman from Oklahoma who developed a rare form of glioblastoma multiforme at the age of 44. Mike was a recipient of the "Profiles in Courage" award and his many achievements are outlined in Caroline Kennedy's book, *Profiles in Courage for Our Time*. Mike was treated at the National Cancer Institute in 1995 and died six months after his diagnosis. To this day, Mike's father, Edmond Synar, remains one of my dearest friends. As a staunch advocate for clinical research and particularly for the National Institutes of Health, Mike Synar would have been thrilled to see the advances in medicine that have improved the quality of life and survival for so many Americans with malignant brain tumors.

Finally, I am thankful for the love that God has for me and for His children, some of whom I have been privileged to know as they spent their last months on earth. I look forward to the time when I will see them again and rejoice in His presence.

Virginia Stark-Vance, MD
Dallas-Fort Worth, Texas
April 2003

Sometimes it is difficult to believe that in June of 2000 I was diagnosed with a malignant brain tumor yet today I am cancer free. There were many days, weeks and months of pain, frustration, and depression, but there have also been so many more days of joy and appreciation for what I have been given that might not have come to me if I had not been challenged with this test of my faith and strength!

My life has not been the same since; I had hoped that someday I would be able to make a difference in other's lives by sharing my story with patients and caregivers that are fighting to overcome brain cancer. Over the last few years, my husband and I have tried to educate ourselves as much as possible about brain cancer; however, I soon discovered just how difficult it was to navigate the ever-changing landscape of cancer information—especially with respect to brain cancer. It also became quite clear to me that brain cancer does not get as much attention as it deserves. When I was asked to coauthor this book and share my personal experiences with brain cancer, I couldn't wait to begin. My hope in writing this book is that you will find in it the answers that will assist you in asking the questions the next time you go to the doctor, and that you find the strength and encouragement to help you cope with the personal sadness or difficulties that you or a loved one may be experiencing. We have a common experience and perhaps I might provide some insight into what you may be searching for.

This book is dedicated to the many people who have touched my heart in so many ways and given me the courage and inspiration to live each day to the fullest and to never take life for granted. First, to my husband, Duane, who is the love of my life and is my constant source for strength, confidence and perspective. Initially we thought we might lose each other... but with communication and education we both came to realize that brain cancer is not a death sentence. In fact, it is an *opportunity* to understand that life is finite and you must live each moment to its fullest. Only those that are in this situation can understand this, and it is you to whom I'm reaching out. I don't know what I would do without him by my side every step of the way. To my parents, Ruth and Dennis Coughlin, who taught me to never be afraid to take a challenge and to take charge of my life. They also instilled in me a sense of humor that has allowed me to keep life in the proper perspective. I am also grateful to the rest of my family who taught me how to be strong and were there as "my rock" when I found it difficult to be strong. I am extremely thankful to so many others who provided constant support, encouragement and lots of humor to get me through the toughest of times including Cissie Wagner, Beth and Bill Conner, Jayne and Gil Romo, my pastor Father Henry Petter and all of the members of my church and extended family who prayed daily for my recovery.

I am especially thankful for the doctors, nurses, and support staff at Baylor Richardson Cancer Center who became more like family than a medical team. I am grateful to my co-author, Dr. Virginia Stark-Vance who had the confidence in my abilities to write this book with her. Writing this book took more time and research I think than either Dr. Stark-Vance or I anticipated when we first began. I still do not know how she managed to fit this book in to her busy schedule of driving back and forth from Dallas to Fort Worth just about every day, making rounds at several hospitals, spending the night at the hospital where she made rounds and also managed to see patients in each of her two offices... all the while attempting to have some sort of a personal life. She continued to encourage me to share my personal experiences in an effort to help other brain tumor patients and caregivers recognize that they were dealing with the same fears, frustrations and uncertainties that I was. Dr. Stark-Vance started out as one of my doctors but has become a trusted friend and advisor. I would also like to thank our editors, Elizabeth Platt and Chris Davis at Jones and Bartlett Publishers. They not only believed in this book but were constantly providing the support that was needed while affording us the latitude to include additional information that Dr. Stark-Vance and I felt was imperative for the readers of this book to know. And to the many other people whose names ought to be here but aren't, please know how significant your comfort and inspiration has been to me.

Finally, I am most thankful for the many blessings I have received and continue to receive from God, and I trust that you will be on the path to getting well... very soon.

M.L. Dubay
Plano, Texas
May 2003

PART ONE

The Basics

What is a brain tumor?

Why are there so many different
types of brain tumors?

Can any part of the brain have a brain tumor?

More ...

1. What is a brain tumor?

The human brain is usually thought of as a single organ, a living computer that receives information from the senses and directs responses to our internal organs and muscles. Actually, the brain is only one part of the **central nervous system (CNS)**, which also includes the spinal cord and the **meninges**, the three layers surrounding the brain and spinal cord. Like the other organs of the body, the central nervous system is composed of individual cells. These cells differ in their structure and function, but all have a normal function, directed by **deoxyribonucleic acid (DNA)**, the internal genetic material of the cell nucleus. Occasionally, the genetic material develops a mutation or error that disrupts the function of the normal cell. If this abnormal cell continues to grow, divide, and produce more abnormal cells, the mass of abnormal cells may eventually become a visible tumor. In the brain, an enlarging mass of abnormal cells that have "forgotten" their original function may disturb the surrounding normal cells in several ways:

- The tumor may create pressure on a section of nearby normal brain, pushing the brain against the skull.
- The tumor may obstruct the flow of blood or spinal fluid circulating in the brain.
- The tumor may spread into the spinal fluid, creating more tumors in the brain and spinal cord.

The word "tumor" as used above is not specified as **benign** or **malignant** (noncancerous and cancerous).

Central nervous system (CNS)

the brain and spinal cord.

Meninges

membranes covering the brain and spinal cord.

Deoxyribonucleic acid (DNA)

the genetic information in the cell nucleus, containing directions on cell growth, division, and function.

Benign

not cancerous; not life-threatening.

Malignant

cancerous; cells that exhibit rapid, uncontrolled growth.

For some brain tumors, there is not a perfect distinction between these terms. Although benign tumors are often characterized as slow-growing or unlikely to spread within the brain, some "benign" tumors cannot be removed surgically and, therefore, cause severe disability and death. Other benign tumors appear to develop further genetic damage over time and become even more rapidly growing masses, a process called **malignant transformation**. Malignant brain tumors tend to grow rapidly, damaging normal brain cells in the surrounding area. They may spread into other areas of the brain, spinal fluid, meninges, or spinal cord. Unlike malignant tumors of the breast, lung, colon, and other organs, malignant tumors of the brain rarely spread to other organs of the body. While "benign" tumors can be dangerous, a few malignant tumors can also be cured.

There are over 100 different types of tumors that originate in the brain, the spinal cord, or the meninges. Throughout this book these tumors will be called **primary brain tumors**. However, many cancers originate in other organs of the body and can spread through the blood stream to the brain, forming a tumor that is identical to the original tumor. These tumors are called **metastatic** or **secondary brain tumors**. Some patients have brain metastases many years after the diagnosis of cancer. Some patients have brain metastases even before they know they have cancer.

The Basics

Malignant transformation
the development of more destructive, invasive, or rapid growth in a previously benign or indolent tumor.

Primary brain tumor
tumors that develop from mutations of normal cells originating in the brain, the spinal cord, or the meninges.

Metastatic tumors
cancer that has spread outside of the organ or structure in which it began to another area of the body.

3

2. Why are there so many different types of brain tumors?

To understand why there are so many types of brain tumors, it is necessary to learn some basic facts about normal brain cells. The **neurons** are cells that send electrical and chemical signals to other neurons. They perform the "work" of the nervous system. It is estimated that there are 1,000,000,000,000 (1 trillion) neurons, each with as many as one thousand different connections to other neurons. The **glial** cells, which outnumber neurons nine to one, support the neurons. Some glial cells make myelin, an insulating sheath that allows neurons to conduct electrical signals at high speed. Some glial cells separate groups of neurons from each other, and some line the spinal fluid spaces of the brain. The major types of glial cells include **astrocytes**, **oligodendrocytes**, and **ependymal** cells.

How a normal cell becomes genetically damaged is not known, but the damage apparently causes the cell to divide repeatedly, producing a mass of cells. The most common brain tumor in adults is **astrocytoma,** which is not surprising considering that the majority of cells in the brain are astrocytes. Similarly, abnormal oligodendrocytes that grow into a tumor become **oligodendrogliomas**, and abnormal ependymal cells become **ependymomas**. All of these tumors may be either benign (as the term is used above, slow-growing) or malignant (fast-growing, destructive). The names of many types of brain tumors are derived from their normal cell or tissue of origin, with the addition of the suffix "-oma." For example, tumors involving meninges are called meningiomas, tumors of the glial cells are

Neuron

nerve cell that conducts electrical or chemical signals.

Glial

supportive tissue of the brain; includes astrocytes, oligodendrocytes, and ependymal cells.

Astrocytoma

a glioma that has developed from astrocytes.

Oligodendroglioma

abnormal oligodendrocytes that grow into a tumor.

Ependymoma

tumor that has developed from abnormal ependymal cells.

4

called gliomas, and tumors involving schwann cells are called schwannomas.

3. Can any part of the brain have a tumor? Where do most brain tumors occur in the brain? Are there areas of the brain where it is more dangerous to have a tumor?

Both benign and malignant tumors can occur in all parts of the body, and the brain is no exception. The central nervous system includes the three major sections of the brain—the **cerebrum**, the **cerebellum**, the **brain stem**—and the spinal cord (Figure 1). The

Cerebrum

the largest area of the brain; divided into the right and left cerebral hemispheres.

Cerebellum

part of the brain that controls balance and coordination, affecting movements of the same side of the body.

Brain stem

that part of the CNS responsible for a number of "unconscious" activities, including breathing, heart rate, wakefulness, and sleep.

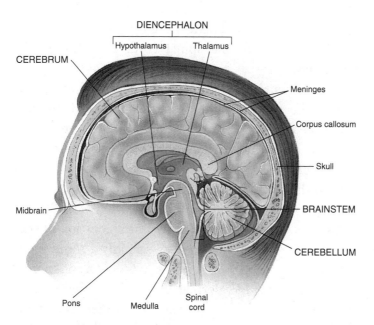

DIENCEPHALON
Hypothalamus   Thalamus
CEREBRUM
Meninges
Corpus callosum
Skull
Midbrain
BRAINSTEM
CEREBELLUM
Pons   Medulla   Spinal cord

Figure 1   The central nervous system, including the three major sections of the brain—the cerebrum, the cerebellum, the brain stem—and the spinal cord. Reproduced from Alters S, *Biology: Understanding Life,* Third Edition. © 2000 Jones and Bartlett Publishers, Inc., Sudbury, Massachusetts.

The Basics

5

Hemisphere

one of the two halves of the cerebrum or the cerebellum.

Corpus callosum

a prominent nerve fiber bundle in the center of the brain connecting the cerebral hemispheres.

Cortex

the outer surface of the cerebral hemispheres; often called the gray matter.

Fissures

the deep folds that separate each cerebral hemisphere into lobes.

Frontal lobe

area of the brain involved in emotion, thought, reasoning, and behavior.

Temporal lobe

area of the brain used for sound, vision, and spoken language.

Parietal lobe

area of the brain that controls sensory and motor information.

Occipital lobe

area of the brain that interprets visual images as well as the meaning of written words.

cerebrum, the largest part of the brain, is divided into right and left **hemispheres,** which connect across the middle at the **corpus callosum.** The outer surface of the hemispheres, the **cortex,** is often called gray matter. It is slightly gray because of the dense population of cells packed into its convolutions (the ridges on the surface). At first glance, the cerebral hemispheres seem to have only a random collection of crevices and bulges, but there are deep folds or **fissures** that separate each hemisphere into lobes. Each cerebral hemisphere is subdivided into the **frontal** lobe, the **temporal** lobe, the **parietal** lobe, and the **occipital** lobe. Directly under the occipital lobe at the back of the head is the cerebellum, which is also divided into two hemispheres. The brain stem is a knob-like structure that is located in front of the cerebellum and under the cerebrum. The lower end of the brain stem is continuous with the spinal cord. Two elongated, curved openings in each cerebral hemisphere, called the **lateral ventricles,** connect with two slit-like openings in the center of the brain, called the **third** and **fourth ventricles** (Figure 2). Spinal fluid is produced in the **choroid plexus,** two spongelike tissues in the lateral ventricles. A tumor can occur in any of these parts of the brain, spinal cord, and meninges.

The symptoms of tumors vary with the location of the tumor. The **grade** influences how rapidly a tumor will cause symptoms. Grade refers to how much the tumor appears to resemble normal brain under the microscope. **Low-grade** tumors typically have few cells that are dividing at any one time. A **high-grade** tumor has a rapid growth rate, and the cells may appear disorganized and distorted. There are, of course, tumors that

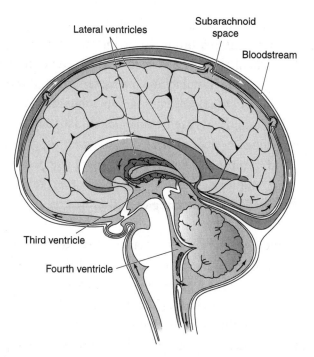

Lateral ventricles

Subarachnoid space

Bloodstream

Third ventricle

Fourth ventricle

Figure 2 Two elongated, curved openings in each cerebral hemisphere, called the lateral ventricles, connect with two slit-like openings in the center of the brain, called the third and fourth ventricles. Illustration adapted from the American Brain Tumor Association.

are somewhere in between these two extremes. These tumors are called **intermediate-grade** tumors.

The cerebral hemispheres direct motor function to the opposite site of the body, but the cerebellum, which coordinates movement, affects the same side of the body. For example, in most right-handed people the left hemisphere controls speech as well as motor function to the right side of the body, so the left hemisphere is considered the **dominant** hemisphere. However, some left-handed people are also considered left-hemisphere dominant because their speech center is located in the left hemisphere.

The Basics

Lateral ventricles

two elongated, curved openings in each cerebral hemisphere connecting with two slit-like openings in the center of the brain.

Third and fourth ventricles

two spinal fluid-filled spaces in the center of the brain in communication with the lateral ventricles.

Choroid plexus

two sponge-like tissues in the lateral ventricles that produce the spinal fluid.

Grade

the degree to which tumor tissue resembles normal tissue under the microscope. Tumors are classified as low grade if they are still very similar to normal cells, high grade if they have a rapid growth rate with distorted or disorganized cells, or intermediate grade if they fall in between low and high grades.

Dominant

ruling or controlling.

The frontal lobes of the cerebral hemispheres govern emotion, thought, reasoning, behavior, and memory. The ability to articulate speech is controlled by the dominant frontal lobe. The parietal lobes control sensory and motor information and the dominant parietal lobe is responsible for understanding written and spoken language. The temporal lobes contain both auditory and visual pathways, and interpret sounds and spoken language for long-term memory. The occipital lobes interpret visual images as well as the meaning of written words.

The cerebellum controls balance and coordination, affecting movements of the same side of the body. The brain stem is responsible for a number of "unconscious" activities, including breathing, heart rate, swallowing, wakefulness, and sleep. Many of the **cranial nerves,** the nerves that provide motor and sensory function to the eyes, mouth, tongue, neck, and shoulders arise from the brain stem. The brain stem is continuous with the spinal cord, with the boundary between the two set at the **foramen magnum,** the large hole at the base of the skull.

Cranial nerves

nerves that provide sensory and motor function to the eyes, nose, ears, tongue, and face.

Foramen magnum

a large hole at the base of the skull that serves as the boundary between the brain stem and the spinal cord.

The cerebral hemispheres make up the largest mass of the central nervous system, and most of the primary brain tumors affecting adults occur in this area. In children, primary brain tumors more often affect the cerebellum and brain stem. Spinal cord tumors are relatively uncommon in both age groups.

The brain stem and cranial nerves are surrounded by the base of the skull, which has numerous small openings for the blood vessels and nerves that travel to and from the brain. However, the space within the skull is limited.

An expanding tumor that exerts pressure on the brain stem may affect consciousness, heart rate, and breathing. Tumors in this area are also more difficult to remove without injuring the normal brain structures and blood vessels. Although all tumors can cause symptoms, tumors that directly or indirectly affect the brain stem are some of the most difficult and dangerous to treat.

4. How common are brain tumors? Is it true that brain tumors are more common in children than in adults?

About 1.2 million adults in the United States are diagnosed with cancer every year, and of those, 35,000 will have a primary brain tumor. Almost half of primary brain tumors are malignant. Primary brain tumors account for only about 2% of all cancers in adults, and with the many different types of brain tumors, some forms are very rare.

In the United States, 8,600 children ranging from birth to age 14 are diagnosed with cancer each year. Brain tumors account for about 20% of all cancers in children (about 1,800 cases). However, the risk of developing a brain tumor increases with age. A person is four times more likely to develop a brain tumor at age 55 than at age 12, and ten times more likely to develop a brain tumor at age 75 than at age 35. The national cancer registry has reported a steady increase in the incidence of brain tumors over the last 20 years, particularly in the elderly population. Part of this increase appears to be related to the improved detection of brain tumors with **computed tomography (CT)** and **magnetic resonance imaging** (MRI) scans.

Computed tomography (CT scan)

computerized series of x-rays that create a detailed cross-sectional image of the body.

Magnetic Resonance Imaging (MRI)

a radiographic study based on resonance from atoms in a strong magnetic field.

The Basics

5. What causes a brain tumor?

Because there are so many different types of brain tumors, each originating from the different types of cells within the brain, spinal cord, or meninges, it is impossible to determine a cause for most brain tumors. There are, however, known risk factors for the development of some types of tumors.

Cigarette smoking has not been clearly associated with an increased risk for the development of primary brain tumors, but smoking is an important cause of metastatic brain tumors, particularly those that originate from lung cancer. Of the 170,000 lung cancer patients diagnosed each year in the United States, about one-third will develop one or more tumors in the brain — more than 55,000 people!

There are some primary brain tumors that affect men more commonly than women and vice versa, but the reasons for these differences are not known. There are also some studies suggesting that workers in certain occupations have a higher incidence of brain tumors. Table 1 lists occupations that have been associated with an increased risk of brain tumors. The increased risk is expressed as an odds ratio (OR). The odds ratio is found by dividing the odds of being in a specific occupation and having a brain tumor, by the odds of being in the occupation but not having a brain tumor. For many occupations studied, there was no known exposure to a potential cancer-causing chemical. Some researchers have suggested that patients with professional or highly paid jobs have better access to medical care, which may result in a greater number of brain tumors diagnosed. However, it is interesting to note

Table 1 Occupations associated with increased risk of brain tumors

Occupation	Odds Ratio	Comments
Statisticians	3.72	Study from New Zealand, 1989
Livestock farmers	2.59	Exposure to animal disease
Truck drivers	6.65	Specifically glioma
Utility workers	13.1	
Printers, publishers	2.8	
Brickmasons	2.5	
French farmers	1.25	Possibly related to pesticide use in vineyards
Petroleum workers	2.9	Not all studies show increased risk
Electrical workers	2.8	Risk increased with exposure to electromagnetic fields
Clergymen	3.8	

that in Sweden, where there is universal access to free medical care, some occupations are still observed to have a higher risk of brain tumors. These include medical professionals, biologists, agricultural research scientists, and dentists.

Patients who have previously had radiation therapy to the brain, skull, or scalp are at risk for developing brain tumors many years later. Several studies have investigated other sources of radiation, such as electromagnetic fields, power lines, and cell phones. However, studies have not yet proven that these sources cause brain tumors.

Head injury, hair dye, and drug use have also been studied, but it has not been shown conclusively that these factors cause primary brain tumors. Food additives and preservatives and chemicals in drinking water have been studied in a number of countries. For example, eating preserved, smoked, or pickled meat and fish appears to correlate with an increased risk of brain tumors. In addition, two studies have shown that the risk of brain tumor decreases when individuals eat more fruits and vegetables. However, other studies of dietary influence on the development of brain tumors have been inconclusive.

In summary, though many factors have been studied for a possible link to the development of primary brain tumors, few are considered definite risk factors.

6. Are brain tumors inherited?

There are some genetic diseases that are clearly associated with the development of specific brain tumors. Fortunately, most of these are rare. Whereas only about 5% of brain tumor patients have a family member with the same or a very similar brain tumor, about 19% of all brain tumor patients have a close family member with another type of cancer. This suggests that the tendency to develop genetic damage that causes abnormal cell growth may be inherited, but the tendency to develop a specific tumor may not be inherited.

Table 2 lists genetic syndromes that have been associated with brain tumors. A brain tumor may contain

Table 2   Genetic syndromes associated with brain tumors

Syndrome	Chromosomal Abnormality	Gene	CNS Tumors Associated with Abnormality
Multiple endocrine neoplasia type 1	11	MEN–1	Pituitary adenoma
Neurofibro-matosis 1	17	NF1	Neurofibromas, optic nerve glioma, meningioma, nerve sheath tumors
Tuberous sclerosis	9, 16	TSC1/TSC2	Subependymal giant cell astrocytoma
Von Hippel-Lindau	3	VHL	Hemangioblastoma
Li-Fraumeni	17	p53	Glioma
Gorlin's syndrome	9	Ptc	Medulloblastoma
Turcot's syndrome	5	APC	Astrocytoma, glioblastoma, Medulloblastoma
Cowden's disease	10	PTEN	Dysplastic gangliocytoma of cerebellum
Pallister-Hall syndrome	7	Gli3	Hypothalamic hamartoma
Rubinstein-Taybi Syndrome	16	CBP	Medulloblastoma, oligo-dendroglioma, neuroblas-toma, meningioma
Familial Retinoblastoma Syndrome	13	Rb	Retinoblastoma, glioma, meningioma, pineo-blastoma

The Basics

13

one or multiple mutations, but that does not mean that the abnormal gene containing the mutation will be inherited by the patient's children. Only those abnormal genes that are present in the reproductive cells (eggs and sperm) are inherited. In many of the syndromes listed, more than one type of cancer has been described. In Turcot's syndrome, for example, all patients who inherit the gene will develop colon cancer if untreated. Because of more widespread genetic testing, many families who are affected by one of the genetic syndromes shown in Table 2 are aware of their increased cancer risk.

Sporadic mutations (those that develop spontaneously and are *not* present in the reproductive cells) account for more than 95% of all brain tumors. However, some of the same mutations described in inherited brain tumors also occur in tumors arising spontaneously. The p53 mutation, for example, is found in over 50% of all human cancers. For reasons that are unclear, younger patients with glioblastoma are more likely to have a p53 mutation than older patients.

M.L.'s comment:

It was June 28, 2000 when I found out that I had a brain tumor. That day was supposed to be just like any other day, but when my alarm went off I woke up feeling like I had the flu, and I just wanted to go back to sleep. I remember I didn't sleep well the night before. I just kept tossing and turning. I felt like I never really went to sleep all night. I hadn't ever had a migraine, much less a headache, but when I finally did get up I knew something wasn't right.

It was 6 a.m. and I was in the shower getting ready to go to work. I remember feeling just awful, as if I were going to faint. My husband, Duane, was out of town, so I couldn't ask him for help, and he wasn't there to see if I was acting strangely. When I got out of the shower all I could think about was how tired I was and that I wanted to go back to bed. I just thought that I needed more sleep because I had worked late at the office the night before.

I called my secretary, Cissie, and told her how I was feeling. She said that I had left her a few notes the night before and she mentioned that they were a bit incoherent (this didn't really surprise me because frequently my notes can be incoherent). Cissie told me that I needed to get some more sleep and that she would take care of everything, so I dried my hair and went back to bed.

When I woke up again it was 9 a.m. and I knew I needed to get to the office. I drove myself to the office because I still thought that I just had the flu or something. To this day I don't remember making that drive. Thank goodness I made it there without getting into an accident.

I arrived at the office around 10 a.m. When Cissie saw me, she knew immediately that something was wrong. At the time, Cissie had been working with me for about four years so she knew me quite well. I was supposed to have lunch with my friend, Beth, that day, and she had already called to confirm our lunch. Cissie knew Beth, and when she called, Cissie had explained to her what was going on with me. Cissie had already asked Beth to come over early because she just had an instinct that something was seriously wrong.

Beth immediately came to pick me up. She took me to the emergency room at the hospital that was, fortunately, just a few blocks away. Once I was in the emergency room, everything became a blur! Later, I was told that I underwent a series of tests, including a CT scan and an MRI. After many tests and lots of questions, the doctors determined that I had an abnormality on the left side of my brain. I was admitted to the hospital and was started on anti-seizure medication. The doctors were concerned that I may have had a mild seizure the night before, and they wanted to prevent a possible recurrence. I remember Beth told me that she had called my husband to tell him what had happened to me. Then she told me to just go back to sleep, which is what I did for most of the day.

Duane was away on a motorcycle trip, but he was only about 5 hours away. Beth told him that I had been admitted to the hospital and that the doctors had found "something on my brain." She told him to get to the hospital as quickly as possible. When he got to the hospital he collapsed at my bedside in tears, terrified that he would never see me the way that I was BEFORE he went out of town. He later told me that he thought I had suffered a stroke. He was so afraid that he would find me lying in bed unable to speak. He also told me that the motorcycle ride to the hospital was the longest 5 hours of his life.

Later that day, the doctors told us that the tests had revealed a mass in the left frontal lobe. It appeared to be a "glial-type" brain tumor. However, they indicated that the tumor was located in an area of my brain where it could be surgically removed.

At this point, it was time to let my family know what had happened to me over the last several hours. Unfortunately, that task was left to my husband, Duane. He immediately called my parents in Knoxville, Tennessee. Although this was extremely shocking news, my father, a retired orthopedic surgeon, and my mother, a former Navy nurse, understood exactly what they had been told. My parents then informed the rest of my family (three older brothers and one older sister), all of whom live in Knoxville. I'm the youngest of five children and I live 1,000 miles away from the rest of the family. I can imagine how difficult it must have been for them.

I was kept in the hospital for a few days. Then I was allowed to go home to "enjoy" the 4th of July weekend. I returned to the hospital the morning of July 6th so that my neurosurgeon could remove the mass in my brain. For the week or so between diagnosis and surgery, I really don't remember too many details. I was probably in some state of shock; however, when my neurosurgeon told me that I had a brain tumor, the reality set in. That was when it became very clear to me that the world as I had known it had changed forever, and my journey of living with a brain tumor began.

The Basics

PART TWO

Diagnosis and Pathology

What are the symptoms of brain tumors?

Why does every doctor I see ask me so many questions about my symptoms, my previous illnesses, and my family history?

What is a neurological examination?

More ...

7. What are the symptoms of brain tumors? Do all brain tumors cause headache?

Brain tumors may be discovered even when they do not cause any symptoms because brain scans are commonly performed in emergency rooms after head trauma. However, the nature and duration of symptoms are important clues to the location of the tumor and sometimes may even suggest the type of tumor present (Figure 3).

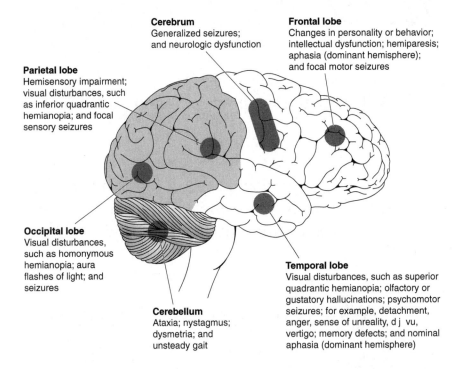

Cerebrum
Generalized seizures; and neurologic dysfunction

Frontal lobe
Changes in personality or behavior; intellectual dysfunction; hemiparesis; aphasia (dominant hemisphere); and focal motor seizures

Parietal lobe
Hemisensory impairment; visual disturbances, such as inferior quadrantic hemianopia; and focal sensory seizures

Occipital lobe
Visual disturbances, such as homonymous hemianopia; aura flashes of light; and seizures

Cerebellum
Ataxia; nystagmus; dysmetria; and unsteady gait

Temporal lobe
Visual disturbances, such as superior quadrantic hemianopia; olfactory or gustatory hallucinations; psychomotor seizures; for example, detachment, anger, sense of unreality, dj vu, vertigo; memory defects; and nominal aphasia (dominant hemisphere)

Figure 3   Signs and symptoms of intracranial tumors. Adapted from *Coping with Neurologic Disorders,* © 1982 Intermed Communications Inc.

It is estimated that, every day, ten million people in the United States suffer from headache. Fortunately, more than 99% of adults who suffer from headache do not have a brain tumor. However, about half of all brain tumor patients complain of headache at the time of diagnosis. Because children seem to suffer headaches less frequently than adults, a child who complains of headache should always raise the suspicion of a brain tumor.

The incidence of headache in brain tumor patients is related to both the growth rate and location of the tumor. Slow-growing tumors are more likely to cause seizures than headaches, whereas faster growing tumors may cause headaches as an initial symptom. Tumors that obstruct the flow of spinal fluid are more commonly associated with headache.

Headaches associated with brain tumors do not always follow a clear, progressive pattern of increasing severity. The headache may be worse in the morning or interfere with sleep, or it may occur with bending, lifting, or exercise. Headaches caused by brain tumors may be relieved with medications used to treat migraine or tension headaches, or even over-the-counter drugs such as acetaminophen (Tylenol) or aspirin.

Other frequent symptoms noted by brain tumor patients include nausea and vomiting, visual problems, seizures, weakness, confusion, imbalance, depression, and fatigue. It is not unusual for family members to note subtle changes in an individual's personality. These changes may be difficult for a doctor to detect unless he is very familiar with the patient. **Neurological deficit** refers to partial or complete loss of muscle

Neurological deficit
partial or complete loss of muscle strength, sensation, or other brain functions.

21

strength, sensation, or other brain functions that may become more pronounced with fatigue. Almost all patients with brain tumors exhibit at least some neurological deficit at the time of diagnosis, although it may be very subtle.

8. Why does every doctor I see ask me so many questions about my symptoms, my previous illnesses, and my family history?

Medical history

a detailed accounting by the patient that helps a physician in determining the length and severity of an illness as well as previous personal and family health history.

A detailed **medical history** is extremely important to a doctor. It helps determine the length and severity of an illness. A patient who comes to the emergency room with a severe headache, for example, may or may not need an emergency CT scan of the brain. Perhaps the patient has a history of migraine headaches for years and has had a normal CT scan in the past. Perhaps the patient fell from a ladder and briefly lost consciousness. Perhaps the patient has had escalating headaches for several weeks that are now unbearable. The doctor must decide, based on an understanding of the patient's complaints, how to direct the physical examination and what tests to order to confirm or rule out a life-threatening condition.

Nonlocalizing

symptoms that don't have a particular location or source. Examples include fatigue, lack of concentration, or nausea.

Localizing

symptoms involving a specific area of the nervous system, such as speech disturbance, weakness of one side of the body, or loss of vision.

Most brain tumor patients have symptoms that may have initially been attributed to other illnesses, depression, or stress. For example, it is common for patients to complain of fatigue, a lack of concentration, or nausea. These **nonlocalizing** symptoms may be easily dismissed by patients and their doctors. **Localizing** symptoms, such as speech disturbance, weakness of one side of the body, or seizures, are more likely to raise the suspicion of a neurological problem.

After taking a careful history, sometimes the doctor can estimate the location of the tumor and its growth rate. The doctor will need to determine whether there is a previous history of cancer because of the possibility of brain metastases. The doctor will also note whether there is a family history of cancer or brain tumor, and whether the patient has other inherited conditions that may impact on the patient's care, such as bleeding disorders, diabetes, and heart disease.

9. What is a neurological examination?

The part of the physical examination called the **neurological examination** actually begins before the patient is aware of it. From the time the patient walks into the examination room, the doctor observes his balance, rhythm, and coordination. During the history, the doctor will observe the patient's speech patterns, whether there is hesitation, difficulty finding words, misuse of words, or slurring of words. Even the patient's eye movements can suggest whether there is a neurological problem.

A neurological examination may be as simple as testing strength, sensation, and coordination in the emergency room setting, or testing a series of more complex physical and memory tasks in the neurologist's office. A complete neurological examination evaluates the following:

1. Appearance and behavior: *Is the patient behaving appropriately for the situation?*
2. Standing and walking: *Is there imbalance or jerking of movement?*
3. Level of consciousness: *Is the patient fully alert?*

Neurological examination

a medical examination testing how well the various functions of the brain are working.

Diagnosis and Pathology

4. Orientation to time and place: *Does the patient know the year, month, day, and where he is at that moment?*

5. General intellectual function: *Does the patient misinterpret clues from the environment or seem confused?*

6. Memory: *Can the patient remember three unrelated words for five minutes?*

7. Speech: *Can the patient understand and respond to spoken language?*

8. Cranial nerve functions:

   I. *Can the patient smell?*

   II. *Can the patient see with each eye separately?*

   III. *Can the patient look up, down, and raise the eyelids?*

   IV. *Can the patient look down and toward the nose?*

   V. *Can the patient open the jaw? Does the patient have sensation on both sides of the face?*

   VI. *Can the patient move the eyes to the right and left?*

   VII. *Can the patient close the eyes tightly and smile symmetrically?*

   VIII. *Can the patient hear with each ear?*

   IX. and X. *Can the patient swallow?*

   XI. *Can the patient shrug his shoulders?*

   XII. *Can the patient stick his tongue out?*

9. Motor function: *Does the patient have normal muscle power in all extremities?*

10. Reflexes: *Are the patient's reflexes symmetrical?*

11. Coordination: *Can the patient touch his finger to his nose rapidly and accurately?*

12. Sensation: *Can the patient perceive light touch, temperature, position, vibration, and pain?*

Some doctors use the **Mini-Mental Status Examination**, which is a set of questions and tasks that can be easily administered in the office or hospital setting. The Mini-Mental Status Examination tests orientation, memory, calculation, language, and figure drawing on a 30-point scale. The test results are kept with the patient's chart to determine whether there has been a change in the patient's status over time.

Mini-Mental Status Examination

a brief verbal and written examination that tests orientation, memory, calculation, language, and figure drawing on a 30-point scale.

10. After my surgery, my surgeon told me that I have a brain tumor but says he can't tell me more about it until the pathology report is completed. What is a pathology report, and why is it so important?

Because there are many different types of brain tumors, your surgeon wants to give you as much detailed information as possible about the kind of tumor you have and the treatment you may need. The doctor cannot do that until a **pathologist** examines the **biopsy** taken at surgery. Some tumors can be evaluated within a few minutes using thin slices of frozen tumor. However, most tumors require processing over a period of several hours. During processing, the water is removed from the specimen. Eventually, tiny pieces of the tumor are embedded in paraffin wax. These small slabs of paraffin-embedded tissue are thinly sliced, placed on microscope slides, and stained with special chemicals that color cell proteins and DNA. These are called permanent sections, and their detail provides the

Pathologist

a physician trained to examine and evaluate cells, tissue, and organs for the presence of disease.

Biopsy

surgical removal of a small piece of tissue or a tumor for microscopic examination.

pathologist with the most complete information about the tumor.

The pathologist provides information about the cells that make up the tumor and identifies whether the cells are native to the brain (a primary tumor) or if they have spread to the brain from another location in the body (a metastatic tumor). The pathologist determines whether the tumor is benign or malignant. The growth rate, or **proliferation index**, can also be obtained from the biopsy specimen using special stains.

In some cases, the pathologist may confer with other colleagues or send the slides to a **neuropathologist,** a pathologist who specializes in the diseases of the nervous system. Difficult cases may take several days of study to determine the exact nature of the tumor. The final diagnosis is written in the **pathology report** (see the Feature, "How to Read Your Pathology Report," on p. 30–31). The importance of this document cannot be overstated. Determining eligibility for clinical trials, the need for further treatment such as radiation therapy or chemotherapy, and the eligibility for insurance or disability benefits are but a few of the reasons why the pathology report is the single most important document to the brain tumor patient (see Question 13).

11. What are the most common types of primary brain tumors?

Table 3 lists the most common types of primary brain tumors in children and adults. In both children and adults, gliomas are the most common type of tumor; however, adults have a higher proportion of malignant, or high-grade, glioma and children have a higher pro-

Proliferation index

a measurement of the growth and division rate of cells obtained from a biopsy specimen using special stains.

Neuropathologist

pathologist specializing in the diagnosis of diseases of the peripheral and central nervous system.

Pathology report

summary of the gross (specimen visible to the naked eye) and microscopic analysis of tissue and/or fluid removed during surgery.

Diagnosis and Pathology

Table 3   Common types of primary brain tumors in adults and children

CNS Tumors in Adults		CNS Tumors in Children	
Glioblastoma multiforme and Anaplastic astrocytoma	35%	Low-grade gliomas and brain stem glioma	44%
Meningiomas	25%	Primitive neuroectodermal tumors (PNET) and medulloblastoma	24%
Low-grade gliomas and brain stem gliomas	12%	Ependymoma	10%
Pituitary adenoma	10%	Pineal region tumors, including germinoma	6%
Acoustic neuroma	7%	Glioblastoma and anaplastic astrocytoma	4%
Other	11%	Other	12%

27

portion of slower growing, low grade glioma. In addition, adults tend to have tumors of the cerebral hemispheres and children more commonly have tumors of the cerebellum and brainstem. Some tumor types, such as primitive neuroectodermal tumor (PNET), medulloblastoma, and ependymoma, are much more common in children; meningiomas are much more common in adults.

12. The surgeon explained to me that I have a fast-growing type of tumor, but I think my symptoms have been present for a long time. Is this possible? Should I get a second opinion from another pathologist to make sure the diagnosis is correct? How do I do this?

It is possible that you have a slow-growing tumor that evolved into a faster-growing type. The pathologist may have only seen the faster-growing component in the tumor specimen studied. Not surprisingly, the treatment recommended for patients with such mixed tumors depends on the more aggressive component.

A second review of your pathology slides can be helpful, but pathologists often confer with others in the same hospital or send the slides to a colleague for further review. It is possible that your slides have been reviewed by a handful of pathologists before the final report is issued. Nevertheless, an additional review—even if the same pathologist does it—may be helpful if you provide clinical information, such as what type of symptoms you have and how long your symptoms have persisted. It is also beneficial if you forward to the pathologist a copy of your MRI.

Getting a second opinion about your pathology slides is particularly important if a different diagnosis will have an impact on your treatment and prognosis. You may ask your surgeon if he recommends sending the slides to another laboratory or research center that specializes in brain tumors. If you plan to participate in a clinical trial, another review of your pathology slides by a neuropathologist associated with the trial is often required.

13. My doctor says that my tumor has a low proliferation index and that I may not need treatment right away. What is the proliferation index, and how does it determine my treatment?

The proliferation index is determined by testing some of the brain tumor sample using a special stain for MIB–1 or Ki–67. The proliferation index is the number of cells involved in the process of cell division (the process that produces new tumor cells) in relation to the total number of cells. Slow-growing tumors have few dividing cells, meaning they have a low proliferation index (sometimes less than 1%). Tumors that grow more rapidly may have proliferation indices exceeding 20%. Tumors with a low proliferation index grow relatively slowly, and even without treatment, they may not appear to have observable growth on an MRI over many months. Tumors with a high prolifer-

How to Read Your Pathology Report

1. The hospital or laboratory that produces the report, usually where the surgery was performed

2. Patient's name, hospital or medical record number, and date of birth

3. The unique number assigned to this case; the reference number to locate slides in the future

4. The surgeon submitting the specimen

5. The impression of the surgeon before diagnosis, often the reason for the procedure

6. The surgeon's notes on the origin of the specimen

7. The final diagnosis may appear before or after the more detailed descriptions of the specimen

8. Preliminary diagnosis by "frozen section" is sometimes helpful to guide the surgeon who must decide if he should attempt to remove more tumor.

9. The dimensions and appearance of the tissue received

10. This is the description of the tumor cells themselves. Key phrases include:
    a. **Infiltrating neoplasm:** Tumor cells that blend into the normal brain without a clear separation.
    b. **Oligodendroglial differentiation:** Based on the descriptions preceding this phrase, the pathologist comments about the probable origin of the tumor. In this case, the evidence suggests that the tumor derived from oligodendrocytes, rather than astrocytes, ependymal cells, etc.
    c. **Focal hemorrhage:** Small collections of blood within the tumor.
    d. **Necrosis:** Literally means dead cells. Often, tumors that have a rapid rate of growth show these areas that have not had sufficient blood supply to allow continued growth.
    e. **Heightened cellularity:** The increased density of cells in a specific area, compared with what would normally be expected.
    f. **Pleomorphism:** Literally means many forms, depicting a variety of cell sizes and shapes.
    g. **Vascular proliferation:** An increase in the number of cells lining the walls of blood vessels of the tumor.
    h. **Mitotic activity:** The activity of cells that are dividing; often seen as dark, irregularly-shaped nuclei.
    i. **Anaplastic:** Growing without structure or form; not resembling orderly normal tissue.

11. MIB-1 staining determines how many cells in a specimen are synthesizing DNA in preparation of cell division; it provides an estimate for the rate of tumor growth.

12. The pathologist who reviews the slides and determines the final diagnosis

St. Mark's Medical Center [1] *
Fordham Ridge, Massachusetts

Doe, John Q. [2]
MR No. 393898882
DOB: 6/26/52
Physician: John Smith, M.D. [4]

Specimen No. S02-887999 [3]
Procedure Date: 7/25/02
Date of Report: 7/26/02

CLINICAL HISTORY: Right frontal brain tumor [5]

DESCRIPTION OF SPECIMEN: Brain, right frontal mass [6]

FINAL DIAGNOSIS: Anaplastic oligodendroglioma [7]

INTRAOPERATIVE CONSULT [8]
An intraoperative consultation with frozen section is diagnosed as marked edema, favor low-grade glioma; defer final diagnosis to permanent sections. Conveyed to Dr. Smith on 7/25/02 by Dr. Jones.

GROSS DESCRIPTION: [9]
Specimen A is received fresh for frozen section labeled "right frontal brain mass" and consists of several soft, tan-gray irregular fragments of tissue which measure 0.8 × 0.4 × 0.3 cm in aggregate. The entire specimen is submitted. Specimen B is received fresh labeled "right frontal brain mass" and consists of a 3.5 × 3.8 × 2.2 cm soft, gray to gray-white wedge shaped portion of brain tissue. The entire specimen is submitted.

MICROSCOPIC DESCRIPTION: [10]
Sections reveal an infiltrating neoplasm dominated by cells with generally rounded nuclei, variably developed perinuclear halos, microcystic change, and a delicate, branching capillary network consistent, in aggregate, with oligodendroglial differentiation. There is focal hemorrhage present, but no frank necrosis is seen. Although much of the lesion appears low-grade, the neoplasm contains areas of heightened cellularity, pleomorphism, early vascular proliferation, and mitotic activity, with up to 2 mitotic figures per high power field, commensurate with an anaplastic (Grade III) lesion. Immunohistochemical stains reveal a moderate to high MIB-1 labeling index, with labeling of approximately 10% of the neoplastic cells in the more active areas, also commensurate with an anaplastic grade lesion. [11]

Dr. Jones and Dr. Brown have reviewed the slides and agree with the final diagnosis.

Signed by: Jane Black, M.D. [12]   Entered: 7/26/02 1530
*Names are fictional throughout

ation index may double in size over a period of a few weeks.

The decision to treat a slow-growing tumor is often based on the type of symptoms that it causes, its location, and the amount of residual tumor present after surgery. For patients who have slow-growing tumors with very little residual disease, the risk of radiation therapy, chemotherapy, and other forms of treatment may outweigh the potential benefit, particularly if the patient does not have symptoms. Your doctor may recommend careful follow-up with MRI and regular neurological examinations.

14. Will my tumor spread to another part of my body? Can it spread to another part of my brain or spinal cord?

Metastatic tumors originate in another cancer of the body, such as the breast, lung, or kidney. They may spread to multiple sites, including the brain. In contrast, primary brain tumors that originate in the brain, such as gliomas, rarely spread to other organs of the body. Some rare primary brain tumors that do metastasize include pituitary carcinoma, hemangiopericytoma, and papillary meningioma.

Primary or metastatic brain tumors may spread throughout the CNS through the spinal fluid, sometimes causing symptoms such as back pain, weakness, or numbness. Leptomeningeal metastases (see Question 49) may be seen on MRI as a coating around the brain or spinal cord. The MRI may also show tiny tumors in the lower spinal cord called "drop" metastases. Some common systemic cancers associated with leptomeningeal metastases include breast cancer, small cell lung cancer, and melanoma. Primary brain tumors that can spread throughout the spinal fluid include primary CNS lymphoma, germ cell tumors, and medulloblastoma.

Some primary brain tumors have multiple sites in the brain at diagnosis and are termed **multifocal**. CNS lymphoma, germinomas, and, less commonly, malignant gliomas can appear at multiple sites in the brain. Biopsy of at least one area is necessary to distinguish between a multifocal primary tumor and a metastatic tumor because treatment recommendations for these tumor types may differ.

Multifocal
having more than one point of origin.

M.L's comment:

I had no idea how important the pathology report was. Although the actual report wasn't reviewed with me, my neurosurgeon did discuss the specifics of it. He indicated that the pathology report revealed that I had an oligodendroglioma. However, after my neurosurgeon received the analysis he sent it back to be retested because he thought that what he removed looked like something other than an oligo. Nevertheless, the test came back again with the same result. Clearly, an accurate diagnosis is extremely important to my neurosurgeon because the recommended treatment hinges on the interpretation of the pathology report. A copy of the pathology report was one of the first documents that I had to send to my disability advisor after my surgery so that I could apply for temporary disability.

PART THREE

Neuroimaging

Why do I need a CT scan and an MRI?

How does MRI work?

I have had surgery and radiation therapy for a brain tumor. How often should I have a follow-up MRI scan?

More ...

15. I had a seizure at work and was brought to the emergency room. I had a CT scan, which was abnormal, but then the doctor also ordered an MRI scan. Why do I need both?

Most patients have both a CT scan and an MRI because they provide different information. Many emergency rooms use CT (computed tomography) scans as an initial screen for tumors, stroke, hemorrhage, and other neurological conditions. CT is more widely available, less expensive, and can be done in a matter of minutes. An MRI (magnetic resonance imaging) scan typically takes much longer and may not be immediately available. Some patients cannot have an MRI because they have metal pacemakers or other metal devices implanted in their bodies. However, MRI does not use x-rays or iodine contrast, which makes it safer for most patients. In addition, MRI provides more detailed, three-dimensional pictures of the brain. These detailed pictures are particularly important when planning surgery.

Sagittal image

an image that divides the brain into left and right and is particularly good at showing tumors in the exact center of the brain.

Coronal image

an image that divides the brain into front (anterior) and back (posterior) and shows best the deeper and more central areas of the brain.

CT scans typically show only a single plane of the brain (an **axial** image). Axial images are slices through the brain that begin at the crown and end at the bottom of the skull. They are useful because right and left hemispheres of the brain are normally mirror images of each other. It is easy to see any distortion of one of the hemispheres with an axial image. Two other types of imaging planes, **sagittal** and **coronal**, are seen only with MRI. A sagittal image divides the brain into left and right, as if divided from the tip of the nose to the center of the back of the head. This type of image is particularly helpful in showing tumors located in the exact center of the brain. Coronal images divide the brain into front (anterior) and back (posterior), and they show the deeper and more central areas of the brain. Each image on an MRI includes other information, such as the thickness of the slice in millimeters, the number in the sequence, and the right and left orientation of coronal and axial images.

The first scans that you have (those that are performed before surgery and before *any* medications are prescribed, including steroids) are very important. These scans may be needed to help determine your treatment, especially if surgery and radiation therapy are being considered. Although many hospitals insist that your scans are the property of the hospital and must be returned, you can and should ask for copies of your MRIs and CTs. Some facilities will charge for copying each sheet of your scans. Other facilities will not charge for a copy as long as it is taken to one of your doctors. With each follow-up scan, you should ask for a copy to be made at the same time as the original. These copies can be taken to your appointments and reviewed by your doctors, but you should keep them in your possession afterwards. Keep all of your scans together, dry and flat (under the bed is ideal).

16. *How does MRI work?*

This is extremely difficult to explain in laymen's terms, but the very name, magnetic resonance imaging, is a brief description of the principle of MRI. Everyone is familiar with magnets and the fact that magnets have a north and south pole. There is a magnetic field of the Earth, but the magnetic force of an MRI in a hospital is at least one thousand times stronger than the Earth's magnetic force. If you imagine that the nuclei of the hydrogen molecules of the brain are magnets, you can understand that they have a north and south pole. In the magnetic field of an MRI unit, all of the north poles of the hydrogen nuclei of the brain align in one direction. The MRI unit sends a radio signal to the nuclei, which causes them to flip 90 degrees. When the radio signal switches off, the nuclei go back to their original position. As the nuclei change position, they emit an electromagnetic signal (resonance) that is captured on a computer. The computer determines exactly where the signal is coming from, and it is this localization that produces an image. The strength of the electromagnetic signal from abnormal tissue in the brain is different from the signal from the normal brain, producing a different shade of gray or different **radiosignal**. Most patients suspected of having a tumor will be given an intravenous injection of a chemical agent called gadolinium. The gadolinium makes the blood vessels distinctly white against the gray background of the normal brain. Some tumors will also show bright areas of enhancement when gadolinium contrast is used.

Although it is an oversimplification to say that MRI detects the subtle differences in the hydrogen content of the structures of the brain, that's exactly what it does. All of the clicks, buzzes, and banging that you hear during an MRI examination are circuits causing the magnets of the hydrogen nuclei to flip back and forth. A typical MRI scan includes several different types of images. Each image provides different information. Your doctor will specify whether you need an intravenous injection of contrast and whether special views or thinner slices are required.

Radiosignal

in MRI, the image produced by resonance of hydrogen atoms in a magnetic field during and after a radiofrequency pulse.

M.L.'s comment:

I have had a lot of MRI scans (over a dozen now), and although I'm not claustrophobic, I can see why a lot of people would have a difficult time with an MRI. Lying on a table and having this machine slide you in to what feels like a very cramped tunnel can make anyone feel like they need to get out! One technique that seems to work for me is to close my eyes and take deep breaths. I focus on the breath that I'm taking in and the one that I'm breathing out. I try not to think about the fact that I'm in a "tunnel." By using this technique, I usually come pretty close to falling asleep, especially because my medication makes me kind of sleepy anyway. Also, make sure that the MRI technician gives you some earplugs. The MRI machine can be kind of loud. The earplugs really help cut down on the noise, and sometimes they make it easier for me to fall asleep. When the technician gives me the contrast dye, I try not to let it get to me, but I just don't like being stuck with needles. So far, I've been pretty lucky and haven't had anyone hurt me. Typically, those that have to take blood or give contrast dye on a regular basis have the procedure down so well that they know how to do it so that it doesn't really hurt. I NEVER look at the location where the needle is being stuck; I just always make sure and tell the technician, "Please don't hurt me!"

17. I had surgery and radiation therapy for a brain tumor. How often should I have a follow-up MRI scan?

Your doctor considers many factors when determining the frequency of follow-up MRI scans. Although there are no specific guidelines for the follow-up of brain tumors, a general rule is that if the result of the scan would impact on the patient's decision for further therapy, a scan is recommended.

Neuroimaging

How to Read Your Own MRI Scans

Patients who have been diagnosed with a brain or spinal cord tumor are usually carrying around a huge x-ray file folder of their films to their **neurosurgeon** (see Question 23), radiation oncologist, or neuro-oncologist for months before they figure out that these films are, literally, the key to their future. A neuroradiologist can look at someone's brain MRI and predict what will happen next. For example, a neuroradiologist can tell if the patient's right leg will become weaker, if part of the patient's visual field will be lost, and if the patient will develop speech problems. Of course, most neuroradiologists do not actually see the patient. It is up to the doctor taking care of the patient to use the information provided by neuroradiologist to make a treatment plan that will prevent further disability.

Neuroradiologists are doctors who have been trained in general radiology (interpreting a variety of images) and receive further training in the interpretation of images of the brain and spine. Neuroradiologists typically see thousands of brain tumor cases during their training. This experience gives them a unique advantage over most other radiologists and even other neurological aspecialists. However, learning some of the basic principles of MRI interpretation can be helpful to the patient (and almost every brain tumor patient has sneaked a peek at the new scans when given the opportunity).

If an MRI of your brain has already been done at another facility, bring it with you when you have a new scan, even if it is several months old. A neuroradiologist looks for *changes over time*. If your doctor is ordering an MRI scan now, even though you had one three months ago, it is because he is expecting that there are or could be changes in the appearance of the brain in the interval.

Secondly, a neuroradiologist looks for *changes in symmetry* (Figure 1). The tumor or swelling around the tumor may have created a distortion of the center line of the brain called *midline shift* (Figure 2). If the distortion involves compression against another section of the brain, this is called mass effect.

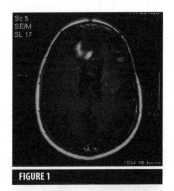

FIGURE 1

Third, you have noticed that MRI scans are black and white images, and their interpretation depends on what can be subtle *changes in gray scale*, reflecting *changes in radiosignal.* Black and white photographs have negatives, but MRI scans are not positive and negative images in the same sense. Although there are often several different kinds of images included in a complete MRI study of the brain, the T2-weighted (or T2 scans) and T1

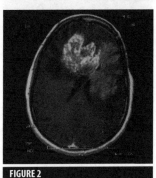

FIGURE 2

weighted gadolinium-enhanced images (often marked with adhesive labels stating the brand of contrast agent used) are among the most important.

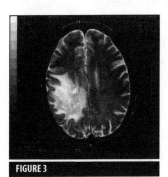

FIGURE 3

Figure 3 is a T2-weighted axial image. This type of image shows the spinal fluid and any excess water in the brain as white. **Edema** (swelling) around a tumor may be very striking, as in the image here. Remember that your symptoms can be caused by this edema, which is why your doctor usually studies these images carefully. However, even when the tumor has been completely removed, there may still be a lighter margin around the area of the surgery for several months because T2 scans are so sensitive to residual water. There are some types of tumors, including some low-grade gliomas, that are detected only on T2 scans. Effects of radiation therapy can also show changes on T2 scans. Many other changes within the brain, including strokes, multiple sclerosis, and infection, can also cause changes on T2 scans.

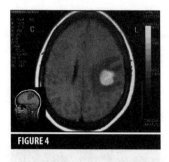

FIGURE 4

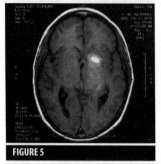

FIGURE 5

Figure 4 is an axial image of a primary central nervous system lymphoma after an intravenous injection of gadolinium contrast. The tumor is much more obvious with contrast because it has caused what neuroradiologists refer to as "breakdown of the **blood-brain barrier.**" In other words, the presence of the tumor has created tiny leaks in the very fine blood vessel networks in the tumor. However, other abnormalities of the brain can also show this dense whiteness, including the changes that occur at the margin of the tumor after surgery. For this reason, many neurosurgeons feel that MRI can be misleading in judging how much tumor remains following surgery. Also, a dense area of white may appear in the brain even before contrast is given, which corresponds to recent bleeding within the brain (Figure 5).

Finally, one of the most difficult changes that a neuroradiologist must detect is *changes that occur as a result of therapy.* Most of the time, a neuroradiologist does not know what therapy has been given. For example, a dense, white area on the scan of a patient who has received radiosurgery may be a recurrent, growing tumor or may be dead tumor **(radiation necrosis).** It can be impossible to tell the difference without a biopsy, although under certain circumstances **positron emission tomography (PET)** can be helpful in discriminating between them (see Question 20).

Figure 6 is the T2-weighted axial image of a patient who has an oligodendroglioma that was first diagnosed by biopsy 10 years ago. This image demonstrates abnormal increased brightness corresponding to increased radiosignal in the left occipital lobe. Notice that there is little distortion or mass effect on the adjacent brain structure. These changes of increased radiosignal, without significant distortion of the

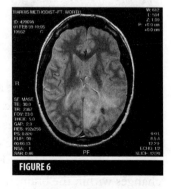

FIGURE 6

adjacent brain structures, are consistent with a low-grade tumor.

Figure 7 is the contrast-enhanced image of a patient who has a malignant glioma that was diagnosed two years before this scan was performed. The tumor causes a distortion of the normal structures of the brain, with both prominent mass effect on the lateral ventricle and midline shift from right to left. After the administration of gadolinium contrast, there is marked increased radiosignal within the tumor. Although the tumor originated in the right frontal lobe, it has now crossed the corpus callosum and extends into the left frontal lobe.

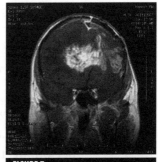

FIGURE 7

Figure 8 is the T1 weighted, contrast-enhanced view that demonstrates multiple abnormalities distributed throughout several lobes of the brain. In this patient with a known history of lung cancer, the

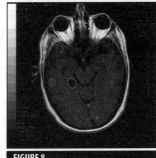

FIGURE 8

abnormalities depicted are most consistent with metastatic lung cancer. Virtually all metastatic tumors enhance with contrast.

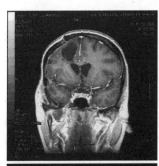

FIGURE 9

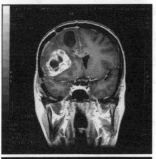

FIGURE 10

Finally, it is unfortunate, although not uncommon, that tumors that have been changing slowly, if at all, on MRI scans may rapidly recur, even over a few weeks. Figure 9 is a T1-weighted, contrast-enhanced coronal view of a patient who has undergone previous surgery for an oligodendroglioma of the right frontal lobe. Eight weeks later, the same area shows that the tumor has recurred as a more aggressive, high-grade glioma (Figure 10). Remember that even relatively subtle changes on an MRI may indicate that a change in therapy is indicated, and these changes may be detected only by performing MRI scans at regular intervals.

MRI scans are often obtained after surgery and several weeks following the completion of radiation therapy. If there is residual tumor present on your MRI scan following radiation therapy, your doctor may order an MRI scan 2 or 3 months later to determine whether the tumor appears to be stable. If there is clear evidence of tumor recurrence over that period of time, your doctor will discuss with you possible treatment options. On the other hand, if the residual tumor appears to be stable or improving, your doctor may continue to monitor your progress with both regular neurological examinations and MRI scans.

Patients on clinical trials always have regular evaluations to determine the success of their treatment, often with measurements of tumor growth or shrinkage on MRI. Patients receiving chemotherapy will also have reassessment on a regular basis, but this may be determined by the cycle length of the drug (see Question 43).

Patients with slow-growing tumors may have follow-up MRI scans every 6 to 12 months. Patients with new symptoms may require follow-up MRI scans more frequently, sometimes as often as once a month, until it is determined whether tumor growth, edema, radiation necrosis, or another factor is responsible for the change.

18. After my surgery two years ago, I have had MRI scans regularly that have been stable. My most recent scan shows a new abnormality near the location of the

original tumor. What are the chances that this is a new tumor? How can I find out?

Not every "new" area on an MRI scan of a brain tumor patient is a recurrence of the tumor—although the possibility of recurrence must be taken seriously. Some other abnormalities that may appear on an MRI scan include radiation treatment effects, vascular abnormalities including stroke, and "artifacts." Artifacts are false images that may be produced by the imaging process or by the movement of the patient. The neuroradiologist interpreting the scan compares all of the images in the series, including the coronal, axial, and sagittal sequences, to determine whether the "new" area is an artifact. However, it is not always possible to tell whether the new area appearing on the MRI is clearly related to the original tumor, particularly with a small abnormality.

Review of the scans with your neurosurgeon may be helpful. He may recommend a follow-up MRI within 4 to 6 weeks to determine whether the abnormality is stable. Although a biopsy could be performed to determine whether the area seen on MRI is a tumor, this would obviously involve more risk. Some abnormalities remain stable or even resolve completely over a period of a few weeks.

19. My neurosurgeon said that I have a "butterfly glioma" based on my MRI. How is this different from any other type of glioma?

A "butterfly" glioma is most frequently a malignant glioma, but the "butterfly" description means that the tumor has crossed over the midline of the brain to involve both the right and left hemispheres. The tumor often appears symmetrical, like the wings of a butterfly. Other types of tumors, however, may also cross the midline to create a "butterfly" appearance. A biopsy is necessary to confirm whether the tumor seen is a glioma or a different type of tumor. Because the tumor involves both hemispheres, it cannot be completely removed; however, some neurosurgeons will try to remove the larger portion of the tumor if it is creating pressure on the surrounding brain.

20. What is a PET scan? Should I have one? Why does my doctor use MRI scans and not PET scans to evaluate my tumor?

Positron emission tomography (PET) is an important imaging tool for many types of cancer and many types of central nervous system disease. Whereas CT and MRI scans reveal the structure (anatomy) of the body, PET scans reveal the differences in living tissues (physiology). PET scans require the administration of a radioactive substance, often a radioactive sugar, such as fluoro-deoxy-glucose (FDG), produced in a cyclotron. There are several radioactive elements that can be used in PET scanning, and they all have an atomic nucleus that undergoes transformation from a proton (a positively charged subatomic particle) into a neutron (a neutral subatomic particle). As a result of this transformation, a positron is released. The positron then combines with an electron, which produces energy in the form of gamma rays. The PET scanner detects the energy formed from the gamma rays, which is then reconstructed to form an image. PET images (see Color Plate 1) do not have the fine detail of MRI scans, but they do show differences in the metabolism, or use of energy, by the brain's cells.

More than 50 years ago, scientists discovered that glucose is taken up by living cells, and that rapidly growing cancer cells take up more glucose than normal cells. Although early studies using PET suggested that the radioactive tracer FDG correlates with the rapid reproduction of cancer cells, more recent studies suggest that there is a correlation between the number of living cancer cells present. However, other conditions, such as infection, may also take up radioactive glucose at higher rates than normal tissue; thus, high FDG uptake does not necessarily indicate cancer.

The difference in uptake of FDG in normal brain tissue and in slower-growing tumors may be slight. Therefore, PET has been used to differentiate between malignant or aggressive tumors (which show more intensely in the scan, indicating more radioactive tracer in this area) and more slow growing tumors (which can show about the same amount of radioactive tracer as the normal brain). Prior to treatment, higher rates of FDG uptake in brain tumors have been shown in some studies to be associated with a poorer prognosis. Following radiation treatment, FDG-PET can be used to distinguish between residual living tumor and tumor that is dead but still shows contrast enhancement on MRI or CT (Color Plate 1).

There are some limitations, however, in using PET to monitor the patient's response to brain tumor therapy. Following therapy, many patients have both tumor necrosis and residual, living tumor present in the brain.

Neuroimaging

A PET scan that shows high FDG uptake suggests there is living tumor present, but a low FDG uptake does not mean that the brain is tumor-free. Small amounts of living tumor could be present.

21. What is magnetic resonance spectroscopy? What does it tell my doctor about my tumor that the MRI does not?

Magnetic resonance spectroscopy (MRS)

a study similar to conventional MRI that measures chemical compounds within the brain.

Magnetic resonance spectroscopy (MRS) is a technique similar to conventional MRI that measures chemical compounds within the brain. Although conventional MRI detects differences in brain water, MRS techniques suppress brain water so that other compounds such as choline, creatine, and N-acetyl aspartate (NAA) can be detected. Detecting these compounds produces a chemical waveform or spectra in a tumor that can be compared to the spectra of an area of normal brain in the same patient. The amount of each of these compounds present in an area of the brain that appears abnormal on conventional MRI can suggest not only the presence of a tumor, but also the grade of tumor and whether necrosis is present. For example, because NAA is associated with living, normal neurons, a *reduction* in the NAA peak reflects an absence of neurons. On the other hard, the choline peak on an MRS is typically *higher* in brain tumors than in normal brain because choline is associated with cell membrane metabolism and dense, rapidly proliferating tumors. Creatine, the third compound, may be either lower or higher than the choline peak in a brain tumor. Areas of necrosis may reveal a fourth peak on an MRS that corresponds to lactate.

Color Plate 2 is an MRS image and its corresponding waveform from an area of a tumor and the area of the normal brain in the opposite hemisphere. The wave-form or spectra from each location reveals the propor-tion of NAA, creatine, and choline present in the tissue. These proportions are clearly different for the two areas, and radiologists who interpret MRS use this informa-tion to detect whether the abnormal areas are more likely to be tumor or necrosis (dead or dying cells). The changes in the spectra can also be evaluated after ther-apy to determine whether viable tumor remains.

MRS has some advantages over PET in that it uses available MRI technology and does not require the use of contrast or radioisotopes. It can be repeated a num-ber of times without risk to the patient. However, MRS has some limitations. MRS may be difficult to interpret in areas of the brain adjacent to the skull. The resolution of an MRS scan is relatively poor, mak-ing it unsuitable for the detection of small abnormali-ties. Like other imaging modalities, MRS cannot reliably differentiate between different tumor types and grades, although future developments in MRS may increase its accuracy. Using several imaging modalities together can give an improved view of the tumor, as in Color Plate 3, which shows MRS used in conjunction with MRI and PET.

22. I have read that functional MRI can show the parts of the brain that control movement and speech. Do I need a functional MRI before my surgery?

Functional MRI, like conventional MRI imaging, detects differences in the magnetic properties of brain tissue, blood vessels, and spinal fluid. In addition, func-tional MRI detects changes in red blood cells and capil-laries as they deliver oxygen to "functioning" parts of

Neuroimaging

Functional MRI

a type of MRI that detects the changes in red blood cells and capillaries as they deliver oxygen to "functioning" parts of the brain.

the brain. For example, although it would be easy to assume that the entire brain is involved in complex activities such as speech, there are in fact very discrete areas of the brain that produce spoken language. These areas actually have higher blood flow and higher oxygen consumption when a person speaks. Functional MRI can detect these subtle but definite differences in oxygen consumption. A map of some of the functions of the brain can be developed by asking the patient to perform specific tasks, such as finger tapping, reading silently, or looking at pictures during an MRI (Color Plate 4). Obviously, some of the more interesting, unique talents that people have, such as artistic or musical ability, are impossible to map on functional MRI.

Functional MRI for localizing certain brain areas before surgery may be useful. For example, a left-handed patient may have a tumor in the left frontal lobe that seems to extend into the area involved in the production of speech. Language dominance in most right-handed individuals is centered in the left hemisphere, but in some left-handed patients language dominance is in the right hemisphere. A functional MRI can quickly and accurately determine the area of the brain involved in speech when the patient silently performs a series of word recognition tasks. This may guide the neurosurgeon around the area (if the speech area localizes on the left near the tumor) or may give him the reassurance that he will avoid it completely (if it localizes to the right hemisphere, opposite the tumor).

Functional MRI is not yet widely available, and there are relatively few situations that require preoperative assessment with it. If your neurosurgeon believes that functional MRI may be helpful in planning your surgery, he may discuss this with you.

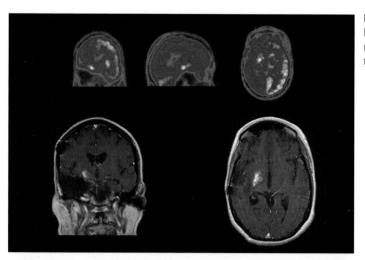

Plate 1. PET/MRI showing both low intensity at the site of radiotherapy and high intensity at the site of recurrences..

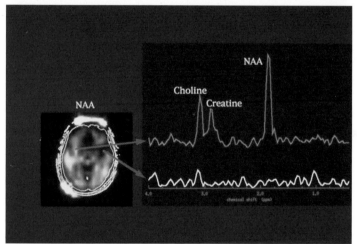

Plate 2. MRS spectroscopy.

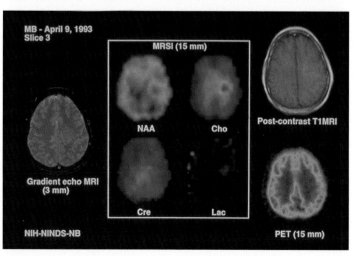

Plate 3. MRI/MRS/PET scanning.

Plate 4. Functional MRI. The spots of color in the image show regions of high uptake.

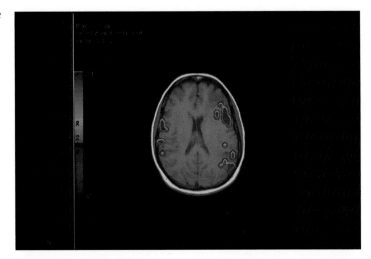

Plate 5. Intraoperative MRI using BrainSuite® imaging technology. Photo courtesy of BrainLAB Inc. BrainSuite® is a registered trademark of BrainLab, Inc. in Germany; registration pending in the United States.

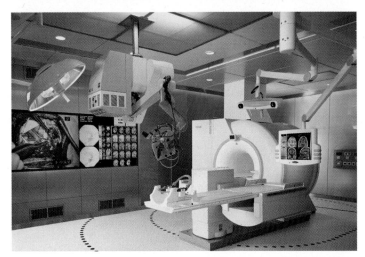

Plate 6. Computer-generated image of an area in the brain to be treated with radiotherapy (RT). Such images are used in planning RT treatment. The colors represent the target area (in red) and relative doses of radiation away from the target (yellow, pink, green, and blue lines).

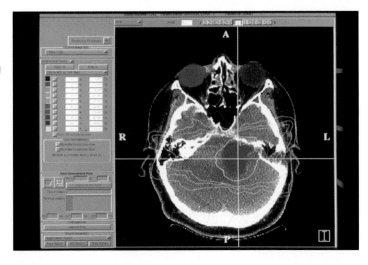

PART FOUR

Neurosurgery

Is surgery necessary to diagnose a brain tumor?

What are the potential complications of
a neurosurgical procedure?

Should I get a second opinion before
having an operation?

More ...

23. Is surgery necessary to diagnose a brain tumor?

Although a brain scan can show an abnormality that looks like a tumor, the only way to determine whether the abnormality is a tumor is by examination of a sample of the abnormality under the microscope. Although there are many ways to obtain a sample of a suspected tumor, with rare exceptions, all of them involve some type of surgery.

Surgeons who operate on the brain and spinal cord have several years of specific training and are called **neurosurgeons.** A neurosurgeon interviews the patient, examines the medical records and scans, and then discusses with the patient the approach to determining the diagnosis. A neurosurgeon usually recommends one of two approaches: a **biopsy** or a **resection**.

A biopsy is removal of a piece of the tumor that will be examined by a pathologist. An **open biopsy** involves removing a small amount of the tumor by carefully cutting through the scalp, skull, meninges, and the brain over the tumor. A **stereotactic biopsy** is the removal of a small piece of the tumor using computer guidance. Often the procedure involves placing a thin needle through a tiny opening in the scalp and skull. The neurosurgeon will decide which of these procedures is the most appropriate for the patient, depending on many factors.

Some patients have tumors that can be completely removed in a procedure called **gross total resection**. If only part of the tumor can be removed because of its size or location, the neurosurgeon may perform a **par-**

Neurosurgeon

a surgeon who specializes in surgery of the central nervous system.

Biopsy

removal of tissue for examination under a microscope.

Resection

surgical removal of a tumor.

Open biopsy

procedure allowing a neurosurgeon to directly visualize the surface of the brain prior to removal of a piece of a tumor.

Stereotactic biopsy

removal of a small piece of the tumor using computer guidance, often with a thin needle placed through a tiny opening in the scalp and skull.

Gross total resection

removal of all visible portions of a tumor.

tial resection. Removal of all or part of the tumor provides enough cells for the pathologist to examine under
the microscope. When neurosurgeons describe a tumor
that can be safely removed, they refer to it as **resectable**.

An open biopsy or resection that removes a part of the
skull is called a **craniotomy**. In most cases, the opening
in the skull is replaced with the section of bone that was
removed to obtain the sample of the tumor. In a few
cases, metal mesh or another type of material is placed
over the brain if the bone must be removed permanently.

There are a few instances that do not allow the examination of a piece of the tumor to confirm the diagnosis. Tumors in the brain stem or spinal cord may be
difficult to biopsy because of the risk of damage to the
blood vessels or normal structures nearby. Metastatic
brain tumors that have spread from another cancer,
such as a lung or kidney cancer, may be removed if the
neurosurgeon determines that the patient will benefit
from its removal. Not all metastatic tumors require
biopsy to confirm the diagnosis if the patient has
already had a biopsy that determined the origin of the
tumor. Finally, a few tumors, such as germinoma or
primary central nervous system lymphoma, may be
diagnosed without surgery if there are tumor cells
present in the spinal fluid. Such patients may have a
sampling of spinal fluid taken during a **spinal tap** or
lumbar puncture. In all cases, remember that a biopsy
is needed to confirm diagnosis so that an appropriate
treatment can be determined.

Sometimes tumors are found that appear to grow
very slowly and have few—if any—symptoms. In
these cases, a biopsy can be delayed for months or

Neurosurgery

Partial resection

removal of some, but
not all, of a tumor.

Resectable

able to be surgically
removed.

Craniotomy

a surgical "cutting" of
an opening into the
skull.

Lumbar puncture

method of obtaining
a sampling of spinal
fluid from the space
between the lumbar
vertebrae (also called
spinal tap).

years. In the unusual circumstance that the patient is too ill to have any form of treatment, a biopsy may not be recommended. The neurosurgeon is trained to make an appropriate evaluation of the patient's circumstances and will recommend surgery only if absolutely necessary.

24. What are the potential complications of a neurosurgical procedure?

The neurosurgeon will discuss with you the potential complications of the procedure he recommends. Although a biopsy may remove a smaller piece of the tumor than a gross total resection, either procedure can be technically difficult depending on the size and location of the tumor. Like all surgical procedures, the possibility of bleeding, infection, and pain will be discussed with you. In many cases, the risks of the procedure can be minimized with careful planning and preparation.

Nondiagnostic

a tissue sample that does not contain adequate information for determining the presence or absence of disease.

For stereotactic or needle biopsies, which remove only a tiny piece of the tumor, the pathologist may determine that the biopsy is **nondiagnostic**. This means that no definite conclusions can be made about the tumor after careful review. In some cases, the small piece of tissue is crushed and the cells are distorted. In other cases, the tumor cells are adjacent to normal cells, and the biopsy needle removes only a sampling of normal cells. There is a higher risk of a nondiagnostic biopsy if the sample removed is very small. If a diagnosis cannot be determined, no treatment can be recommended, and therefore another biopsy must be done. This is extremely frustrating for the pathologist, the neurosurgeon, and most of all, the patient.

More extensive neurosurgical procedures, such as partial and complete resections, may be needed to provide a sample of the tumor to the pathologist as well as relieve pressure caused by the tumor. The difficulty of removing a tumor and the possible risks of removing it depend on multiple factors, including the size and location of the tumor, the blood vessels in and around the tumor, and any previous surgery or radiation therapy performed on the same area. Some elderly patients or patients in poor health may have heart or lung problems that would prolong recovery from surgery. Although neurological functions such as motor strength or coordination may become impaired immediately following surgery, in many cases these deficits resolve with time and with rehabilitation. The risk of seizure following a neurosurgical procedure is low in most patients; however, many neurosurgeons use anti-seizure medication (anticonvulsants) routinely in the postoperative setting.

25. I was taken to my local emergency room and told that I have a brain tumor. The neurosurgeon on call told me I would need surgery right away. Should I get a second opinion before having an operation?

Second opinions can be a good idea. Almost everyone who has to make a serious decision wants to consider all the options carefully. No one wants to feel rushed into a decision about surgery, but there are some tumors that cause life-threatening symptoms or grow so quickly that surgery should be done as soon as possible. As the patient, you need to know whether you have a few days to consider your options or to seek an opinion from another neurosurgeon.

Whenever possible you should speak frankly to your neurosurgeon about your concerns. You should tell him or her that you are considering a second opinion because of the seriousness of the surgery. If your neurosurgeon has done a good job of explaining why you need surgery right away, the type of tumor expected to be found, and whether or not all or most of the tumor can be removed, you should hear similar answers from another neurosurgeon. It is unlikely that two experienced neurosurgeons will give vastly different answers to these questions.

M.L.'s comment:

Regarding a second opinion, my answer would be: it depends. You may not need one or you may not have time to get one. If you've had a seizure and your doctor thinks you may have a glioblastoma, you may not have several days to look for a second opinion. However, if speaking to another doctor makes you feel more comfortable, then you should do so. These days, getting a second opinion is a fairly common practice. In some cases, your insurance company may even require it, especially if surgery is recommended. The most important thing to remember is that you must be sure that it's safe for you to delay your treatment long enough to obtain a second opinion. I was extremely fortunate to have an excellent neurosurgeon. He referred me to other doctors who were also excellent in providing my follow-up care.

26. Are there some brain tumors that can be surgically cured? Is a tumor that cannot be resected always incurable?

Some brain tumors are surgically cured; one of the most common tumors, meningioma, may be completely resected and cured. A number of other tumors, including acoustic neuroma, central neurocytoma, subependymoma, dysembryoplastic neuroepithelial tumor, to name a few, may not recur after complete resection. Some tumors, even if not completely resected, grow back so slowly that another operation may not be needed for many years. Tumors that are completely resected and do not tend to grow back are considered benign. However, benign tumors in certain locations in the brain may still cause death if they cannot be safely removed.

Some tumors cannot be resected surgically; nevertheless, if they respond to other forms of treatment such as radiation therapy or chemotherapy, surgical resection may not be necessary. Germinomas, lymphomas, and other tumors that commonly occur in the deep structures of the brain are often difficult to resect. Fortunately, many can be treated successfully with chemotherapy, radiation therapy, or both.

27. I have seen two neurosurgeons about surgery for my brain tumor, and both say my tumor can be safely removed. One of them says he uses "MRI guidance" to

remove the tumor. What does this mean? Is there an advantage to using MRI to remove the tumor?

Neuronavigation

imaging information that allows the surgeon to localize normal brain structures and tumor.

There are several types of image-guided or **neuronavigation** systems available to assist the neurosurgeon in localizing and removing the tumor during surgery. Some systems use MR images taken before surgery together with special "markers" that are placed on the patient's head. The MR images appear on a computer display in the operating room with the markers still in place corresponding to the exact location on the screen. The neurosurgeon can then use a special pointer to touch areas of the tumor that are seen on the patient's MRI. This allows the neurosurgeon to precisely orient the instruments during surgery, an advantage when the tumor is deep within the brain. Thus, a combination of direct visualization and corresponding MRI imaging may allow the neurosurgeon to remove more of the tumor safely.

Another type of "MRI guidance" is intra-operative MRI (Color Plate 5), which is now available at a few centers. These operating rooms are designed to function with an MRI scanner that can be used during the operation. Also, the neurosurgeon is able to perform a "postoperative" scan while the patient is still on the operating table to make sure the entire tumor has been removed.

Neurosurgeons who use neuronavigation systems and intra-operative MRI may be able to remove tumors that would otherwise be difficult to localize by direct vision alone. In some cases, a more direct approach to the tumor can be planned, reducing the length of the operation and the potential for neurological deficits.

28. One of the people in my support group says that she had "an awake craniotomy" to remove her tumor. What is this procedure, and why did her neurosurgeon do this?

Some patients have a tumor near a critical area of the brain, such as the center that controls speech. Studies such as functional MRI (see Question 22) can demonstrate the location of the speech center before the operation. During surgery, however, many tumors appear to blend into the surrounding normal brain, so it is still possible to damage the speech center when attempting to completely remove the tumor.

In some hospitals and research centers, the patient is allowed to awaken after the neurosurgeon has opened the skull and dura, exposing the brain. The surface of the brain is covered with markers that identify which areas of the brain are involved in the production of speech. The patient may be given a series of words to read during surgery, but if stimulation of an area of the brain shows that the patient can no longer respond, the neurosurgeon knows that removing tumor from this area will most likely damage the speech center.

An awake craniotomy requires more time and preparation for the neurosurgeon and the operating team. Patients who may benefit from awake craniotomy usually have tumors that can be completely resected or will respond to other therapy for any parts of the tumor that must be left behind.

How a Craniotomy Is Performed

A craniotomy ("cranio-" meaning skull and "-tomy" meaning incision) is the process of surgically "cutting" an opening into the skull. A craniotomy may be done for a number of reasons, including repair of a blood vessel, removal of a blood clot, or removal (resection) of a tumor. Performing a craniotomy on a brain tumor patient is not necessarily synonymous with performing a resection. An open biopsy, for example, allows the neurosurgeon to directly visualize the surface of the brain before removing a piece of the tumor. A partial resection involves removing a larger portion of the tumor, and a gross total resection removes the entire visible tumor. All of these procedures begin by first removing enough of the skull to visualize the underlying brain and tumor.

The following account describes what you would see during a craniotomy for gross total resection of a glioblastoma:

Before entering the operating room, the anesthesiologist sees the patient and inserts an intravenous catheter. A sedative is administered and the patient is taken to the operating room. The anesthesiologist and operating room nurses prepare the patient for surgery, placing the patient on the operating table and attaching monitors for temperature, heart rate, blood pressure, and oxygen. The anesthesiologist inserts a hollow tube through the patient's mouth into the trachea that will deliver oxygen throughout the procedure while the patient is asleep.

The neurosurgeon and his assistants position the patient's head in a head holder similar to a vise. The scalp overlying the site of the tumor is shaved and the entire area is scrubbed with surgical soap. The rest of the head and body are covered with sterile surgical drapes.

The neurosurgeon cuts through the scalp with a scalpel, carefully cauterizing small bleeding vessels. The scalp and muscle flap created by the incision are peeled back to expose the skull. The edges of the flap are clamped and covered with a moist sterile cloth. A surgical drill is then placed against the surface of the skull and four bur holes are cut, forming a square. A surgical saw is placed in one of the holes and the four holes are connected, thus allowing a portion of the skull to be temporarily removed. This piece of skull is placed in a sterile salt solution until the end of the operation.

The tough, outermost membrane of the brain, the dura, is cut with scissors to fold back to the edges of the bone, exposing the surface of the brain. The tumor may be visible from the surface of the brain. A deeper tumor may be localized by ultrasound, intraoperative MRI, or another surgical navigation system. The neurosurgeon carefully cuts through the brain overlying the tumor until abnormal tissue is found. This tissue may appear different in color and texture from the surrounding normal brain. The neurosurgeon removes a small piece of the abnormal tissue for examination by the pathologist.

The pathologist prepares the tissue by freezing it in a small block and then slicing it into sections so the tissue can be put onto microscope slides. These tiny pieces of tissue are then stained to reveal the structure of cells. Often, the pathologist can determine immediately whether there is tumor present in the sample, whether the tumor is benign or malignant, and whether it is a primary or metastatic tumor.

If the pathologist is able to make a diagnosis from the frozen section, the neurosurgeon is informed of the result. The neurosurgeon may remove additional pieces of the tumor for further analysis and permanent sections. If the neurosurgeon decides that it is too dangerous to remove additional tumor, the procedure is terminated. However, if the additional tumor can be safely removed or if the removal of large portions of the tumor will reduce pressure on the brain, the neurosurgeon may continue to remove as much of the tumor as possible.

The neurosurgeon and his assistant carefully inspect the brain for evidence of bleeding vessels, cauterizing them and bathing the exposed areas of the brain with sterile fluid. When the neurosurgeon is satisfied that all tumor tissue has been removed and that all bleeding has been controlled, the tumor cavity is filled with a sterile salt solution and the dura is replaced over the brain. The dura is stitched together with suture and checked for any tiny leaks along the suture line. Small holes are drilled through the edges of the piece of skull that was previously removed. This piece is then placed over the dura. Holes are also drilled in the edge of the skull so that suture can pass through both sets of holes to keep the skull piece firmly in place, although some neurosurgeons prefer to use small metal plates and screws to keep the skull piece in position. The muscle and scalp layers are then sutured together, and the free edges of the wound are finally sutured or staped closed. A sterile dressing is then applied to the scalp.

The drapes are removed and the anesthesiologist prepares the patient for awakening. The breathing tube is
removed and the patient is taken to the recovery room.

M.L.'s comment:

*After I finally mustered up the strength to read this section,
it was all I could do to get through it! When I think about
the fact that this was done to me I almost throw up, especially when I read that part about "a piece of my skull is
placed in a sterile salt solution." I also had no idea that the
cavity in my brain where the tumor used to be was filled
up with "sterile salt solution." The part that grossed me out
the most was the description of how everything is "stitched
and stapled" back together. Somehow seeing neurosurgical
procedures on television documentaries isn't quite the same
as imagining that it's happened to your own head!*

29. My neurosurgeon said that if I have a certain type of tumor, he could place Gliadel wafers in the brain after he removes the tumor. But he said that he won't know until surgery what type of tumor I have, and that I have to decide before surgery whether I want him to do this. If I have Gliadel wafers placed during my surgery, can I still have chemotherapy?

Gliadel is a dissolvable wafer impregnated with a
chemotherapy drug called carmustine (also known as
BCNU). The wafer is designed to release chemotherapy
slowly into the surrounding brain to treat microscopic

tumor cells left behind after surgery. Gliadel was developed for malignant glial tumors, particularly glioblastoma, but has also been used for other primary brain tumors. If your surgeon is anticipating, based on your scans, that you have a malignant glioma, he may consider implanting Gliadel after he has resected the entire visible tumor. Gliadel wafers are placed up against the walls of the cavity where the tumor was removed, before closing the membranes, skull, and scalp.

There are some possible side effects of Gliadel implantation. Although very little of the chemotherapy drug enters the bloodstream, it is still possible that chemotherapy leaking into the spinal fluid could affect how the wound heals if the neurosurgeon could not achieve a tight closure of the dura. It is also possible that Gliadel could increase the risk of seizures within a few days of surgery. This can usually be avoided by taking anticonvulsant medication. Finally, a few patients have more swelling of the surrounding brain at the site of the tumor resection when Gliadel has been used.

Gliadel releases chemotherapy into the brain for several days following surgery, but its effects are not permanent. Some patients have continued treatment with intravenous BCNU (the chemotherapy drug that is in the Gliadel wafer) after surgery. While there is theoretically an advantage in continuing to treat any residual tumor cells with BCNU, the intravenous drug—unlike the chemotherapy wafer—affects blood counts and may cause other systemic toxicity. Clinical trials have studied the use of Gliadel followed by other drugs, including temozolomide (Temodar) and CPT–11 (Camptosar). There did not appear to be an increase in the expected side effects with these combinations.

Because Gliadel contains chemotherapy, some clinical trials for brain tumor treatment do not allow patients to participate if they have been previously treated with Gliadel. The patients in a clinical trial must all be similar. The trial results could be difficult to interpret if some patients had received Gliadel and others had not. If it is important to you to enter a clinical trial immediately following surgery, you should discuss this with your neurosurgeon before receiving Gliadel.

However, the randomized trials of patients with glioblastoma who received Gliadel have indicated that long-term survival is improved, and long-term survival may be equal or better than the survival of patients who have had intravenous BCNU. Gliadel is often covered by insurance, but there is also a reimbursement program for patients who do not have insurance. You can find additional information about Gliadel at *www.gliadel.com*.

30. On my most recent MRI, my neurosurgeon told me that my tumor is growing back. I asked him if I should have surgery again, but he told me that he would have to discuss with my other doctors what treatment I could have following surgery. Why does treatment after surgery have an impact on whether I should have a second craniotomy?

As important as surgery is, it may only achieve partial control of the tumor. This is especially true for tumors that spread deep into the surrounding normal brain that are impossible to remove completely. Tumors that cannot be completely removed and grow relatively quickly require other treatments to limit their ability to grow back.

Conventional radiation

radiation therapy delivered by a linear accelerator.

For many patients, **conventional radiation** therapy (see Question 33) cannot be repeated. Therefore, if the tumor grows back after completing radiation therapy, another type of treatment should be used after a second surgery to control any microscopic tumor left behind. If residual tumor is allowed to grow unchecked, the benefit of a second surgery is likely to be temporary.

31. At the time of my surgery, my neurosurgeon said that all of my glioblastoma had been removed, but then he said I would need more treatment to keep it from coming back. Why do I still need therapy if the malignant cells were removed?

Many common tumors, including astrocytomas, oligodendrogliomas, and lymphomas, may appear to be discrete, well-defined masses on MRI. Occasionally, the neurosurgeon will observe a difference in the appearance of the tumor mass and the surrounding brain, but as a rule, these tumors tend to "blend in" and infiltrate the surrounding normal brain. Therefore, the appearance on MRI that the tumor is completely resectable may be misleading. The neurosurgeon may remove all clearly abnormal tissue, but he does not attempt to remove all of the microscopic tumor cells that have spread through the surrounding normal brain. Neurosurgeons who refer to a "gross total resection" are simply referring to their ability to remove all tissue that appeared to be part of the tumor.

Microscopic cells that have spread away from the main tumor mass will continue to grow and must be treated. If the pathologist determines that the tumor is a type that will recur, follow-up treatment after surgery, such as radiation therapy or chemotherapy, is recommended.

32. My neurosurgeon suggested that I have physical therapy and occupational therapy to help me recover from my weakness after surgery. What is the difference between occupational therapy and physical therapy? Do I need both?

Achieving optimal neurological recovery after surgery often means extensive rehabilitation. Rehabilitation programs are available in the inpatient and outpatient settings. Patients may receive rehabilitation while undergoing other therapy such as chemotherapy or radiation therapy.

Rehabilitation programs offer access to a variety of treatment professionals and specialized equipment to help patients receive a structured program for recovery. An initial evaluation by a neurologist specializing in rehabilitation or a **physiatrist**, a physician who specializes in physical medicine, is necessary to identify what should be included in the rehabilitation program. The rehabilitation program is customized to the patient's neurological deficits. Typically, brain tumor patients have a thorough evaluation to identify physical deficits as well as cognitive deficits. Therefore, most patients benefit from a multidisciplinary program.

Physiatrist

physician who specializes in creating rehabilitation programs.

Physical therapy

therapy aimed at recovery from weakness, loss of coordination, or limited endurance.

Physical therapy treats weakness, loss of coordination, and limited endurance. During physical therapy, patients learn to walk unassisted, to use a cane or walker, or to transfer safely from the bed to a chair or wheelchair. Patients may be fitted with a brace or other supportive device to compensate for weak or stiff limbs. Activities may begin while the patient is still confined to bed recovering from surgery because even passive movement of the limbs helps prevent complications such as blood clots and bedsores.

Occupational therapy

therapy that assists patients in relearning activities of daily living such as bathing, brushing teeth, cutting meat, and dressing.

Occupational therapy assists the patient in performing activities of daily living, such as bathing, brushing teeth, cutting food, and dressing. Occupational therapists may use recreational activities such as puzzles to help patients improve their hand-eye coordination and cognitive function.

Other treatment professionals that may be needed in a rehabilitation program include speech therapists, recreational therapists, rehabilitation counselors, and neuropsychologists. Speech therapists evaluate speech production and comprehension. In addition, speech therapists work with patients who have difficulty swallowing. Recreational therapists engage patients in leisure activities, such as cooking, arts and crafts, and music therapy. These activities provide "play" to balance the "work" of physical rehabilitation. Rehabilitation counselors assess the goals of the patient in relation to the return to work and family life. Neuropsychologists specialize in the effect of brain injury on behavior and cognition. They help identify ways to re-learn certain skills as well as advise patients on how to compensate for neurological functions that are impaired.

PART FIVE

Radiation Therapy

What is radiation therapy?

What are the side effects of radiation therapy?

How does the radiation oncologist decide how much of the brain to radiate if nothing is visible on the MRI?

More ...

33. What is radiation therapy? Is radiation therapy given for every type of brain tumor?

Ionizing radiation

a form of energy that knocks electrons out of their normal orbits.

Radiation therapy

treatment that uses high-dose x rays or other high energy rays to kill cancer cells and shrink tumors.

Linear accelerator

a machine used in radiation therapy that is able to create man-made ionizing radiation in the form of x-rays to penetrate through tissue into a tumor.

External beam radiation

the type of radiation therapy delivered by a linear accelerator.

Fraction

single treatment of radiation.

Gray (Gy)

modern unit of radiation dosage.

Centigray (cGy)

unit of radiation, equal to one rad.

To kill a cancer cell, it is necessary to interfere with its ability to grow and divide and form more cancer cells. A form of energy called **ionizing radiation** creates a high enough energy to knock the electrons in the molecules of living cells out of their normal orbits. This creates enough energy to disrupt other nearby electrons, which, in turn, affects the DNA of the cell. Radiation can cause breaks in the strands of DNA, causing cell injury and eventually, cell death. Both x rays and gamma rays are forms of ionizing radiation.

Radiation therapy uses x rays, a man-made form of ionizing radiation, to penetrate through tissue into a tumor. A **linear accelerator** is one machine that produces such radiation. The linear accelerator delivers **external beam radiation** (also known as conventional radiation).

Both normal cells and cancer cells can repair radiation cellular damage to a variable degree. By dividing the dose of radiation into small daily doses called **fractions,** normal cells are relatively spared because they are better able to repair DNA damage. Most cancer cells, however, lack the ability to completely repair DNA damage, and over the course of several days of treatment, the cancer cells will die. The amount of radiation energy absorbed by the body is measured in **Gray**. The amount of radiation used in cancer therapy is typically divided in hundredths of a Gray, called **centiGray,** abbreviated cGy. An older term sometimes used in radiation measurement is the rad, which is equal to one cGy.

Not all brain tumors are treated with radiation therapy, and different types of brain tumors require different radiation **fields** (the volume of brain tissue to be treated). For example, multiple small tumors throughout the brain, which commonly occur in metastatic lung cancer, are usually treated with **whole brain radiation therapy.** This therapy is also used for primary brain tumors that have multiple tumors present at the same time, including primary CNS lymphoma. Most primary brain tumors, which occur as a single abnormality on MRI, are treated with radiation therapy directed at the tumor and a margin of 2 or 3 centimeters around it. This treatment approach is called local, or partial brain, radiation therapy. Sometimes the central portion of the tumor is treated with a high dose of fractionated radiation called a **boost.**

Tumors vary in their **radiosensitivity,** which means that some are easy to control with the standard doses of radiation therapy and some shrink little or none at all. Following surgical resection, some types of tumors will begin to grow back if any microscopic tumor is left behind. Other tumors cannot be removed completely because of their location, and radiation becomes the primary mode of treatment.

Additional types of radiation therapy include **stereotactic radiation** and **stereotactic radiosurgery.** These approaches focus radiation energy to a small area of tumor (usually less than 3 to 4 centimeters in diameter). These therapies do not involve surgery, but they do have "surgical precision."

One type of sterotactic radiosurgery is called **Gamma Knife.** Gamma Knife radiation therapy uses a special

Radiation Therapy

Fields
the volume of tissue to be treated during radiation therapy.

Whole brain radiation therapy
radiation therapy delivered to the entire intracranial contents.

Boost
high dose of fractionated radiation.

Stereotactic radiation
type of radiation therapy that focuses energy to a small area of a tumor, usually less than 3 to 4 centimeters in diameter.

Stereotactic radiosurgery (SRS)
a radiation therapy technique using a large number of narrow, precisely aimed, highly focused beams of ionizing radiation.

Gamma Knife
type of stereotactic radiation designed to deliver radiation from multiple cobalt sources, computer-focused to a small area or multiple small areas.

Cobalt

a radioactive isotope used in the treatment of cancer.

radiation unit that is designed to deliver radiation from multiple **cobalt** sources. A computer focuses the radiation to a small area or multiple small areas. Gamma Knife is most commonly used to treat small metastatic tumors. It may also be used to treat other small benign tumors such as acoustic neuromas, meningiomas, and pituitary tumors. Stereotactic radiosurgery is delivered with one single large dose, 15–30 Gy (ten times the usual daily dose for fractionated radiation therapy). Both Gamma Knife and stereotactic radiosurgery use some type of frame or fixation to keep the patient exactly in position during treatment.

Stereotactic radiotherapy also uses highly localized radiation, but the doses are divided into fractions over a few days. In this case, the frame or fixation used still keeps the patient in an exact location, but can be removed between treatments.

Brachytherapy

radiation therapy that involves placing radioactive material inside the body near or in the tumor.

Brachytherapy delivers radiation therapy from the inside of the tumor to the surrounding area. The radiation can be delivered in several different ways. Sometimes radioactive pellets or seeds are implanted. Sometimes removable sources of radiation are used. Sometimes radioactive liquid is inserted into the tumor cavity or into a balloon catheter that is surgically inserted into the tumor. Gliasite, a balloon device, has recently been approved for insertion into a tumor cavity for the administration of radioactive iodine. Radioactive isotopes have also been linked to monoclonal antibodies to the tumor cells in an effort to more specifically direct radiation therapy to spare normal cells (see Question 39).

M.L.'s comment:

After my craniotomy my neurosurgeon and radiologist recommended further treatment with radiation therapy. Additional treatments with chemotherapy were also recommended, but I didn't start them until after my radiation treatments. Even though my neurosurgeon had indicated that he had been able to remove the entire tumor, it was likely that some cancer cells remained. Those cells needed to be treated with radiation therapy.

The treatments didn't hurt at all. I think the most uncomfortable part of my regular radiation treatments was having the "mask" made for my head and face. I had to lie still—and I mean still—for what seemed like forever while a plastic mesh-like form was molded to my head and face. This was done so that the radiologist could mark in ink the locations where the radiation beams would be targeted every single time that I had a treatment. Before having the technology to make these masks, it's my understanding that the radiologist would make these marks on your skin, and these marks don't just come off with soap and water. Needless to say, the mask is certainly the preferred method, but having to lay still for so long hurt the back of my head a lot more than the regular radiation treatments ever did.

When I refer to "regular" radiation treatments, I'm talking about the daily "conventional" treatments that I received every day for six weeks. I did, however, have additional radiation therapy called stereotactic radiosurgery, but it wasn't the gamma knife procedure. The stereotactic radiosurgery that I received had recently been developed and was called the m3. It was developed by BrainLAB. What the m3 does is allow precisely focused, high-dose x-ray beams to be delivered to a very small area of the brain.

With m3, special planning with the computer allows a large dose of radiation to be delivered to the tumor site with minimal radiation going to the normal or "good" brain tissue that surrounds the tumor site. In my situation, the radiosurgery was delivered as a local "boost" after my 6 weeks of regular or conventional radiation.

This procedure isn't painful; however, you should be prepared for the fact that you have to wear what the doctors call a "halo." It's a metal frame that is placed on your head and attached with screws in four places: two in the back of your head and two in the front. The halo ensures that your head doesn't move during the treatment. The doctors put a topical anesthetic on so that the screws don't hurt too much as the halo is being attached. I also received pain medication, which helped. After the frame was attached, I had a CT scan. The results of that were paired up with the results of the MRI that I had received two days before. By doing this, the medical team that was performing this procedure was able to pinpoint the exact size, shape, and location of the affected area as well as plot the dose of radiation that I would receive that day. The amount of radiation that I received the day of my radiosurgery was almost as much radiation as I would have received during an entire week of conventional treatment. The actual treatment only took about an hour, but the whole process took the entire day because the "planning" procedure took about 6 hours.

I will say that the most painful part was when the halo was removed. I think the pain medication had worn off and when the screws were removed I experienced a terrible wave of pain in my head. It was like having a terrible headache all of a sudden. It didn't last for too long, but that was the only time that the "halo" actually felt more like a "crown of thorns"! If you undergo this procedure, you should make sure that you have been given enough pain medication so that when the halo is removed you don't have to experience the same kind of pain I experienced.

My radiation oncologist said that the headache I experienced after the frame was removed is common. It's caused by a sudden drop in intracranial pressure. You see, the frame produces an intense pressure on the skull, equivalent to 80 pounds per square inch. This pressure on the skull deforms the skull during the hours that the frame is in place. The amount of spinal fluid actually decreases in volume in response to the pressure on the skull. When the frame is taken off, the skull springs back, causing a drop in spinal fluid pressure and a headache. Aside from that one painful moment, I do NOT regret having this procedure because it was the end result that was most important.

34. What are the side effects of radiation therapy?

Several factors influence the risk of developing side effects from radiation therapy. They include the total volume of the brain irradiated, the location of the radiation fields, the total dose received, and the age of the patient. These factors vary from patient to patient.

Radiation side effects may also vary over the course of time. Cells that grow relatively quickly, including those of the skin and hair follicles, are affected relatively quickly, often during the course of radiation. Hair loss in the area of the scalp overlying the tumor is typical.

Patients who receive whole brain radiation therapy may have almost total loss of hair. Hair may grow back for some patients, but for others hair loss may be permanent. Other types of cells, including the normal glial cells of the brain and the blood vessels, are affected months to years after radiation. Occasionally, patients complain of fatigue, weakness, or feeling mentally "foggy" during and for several weeks after radiation therapy. These side effects are quite variable in their severity and duration. Despite these side effects, many patients are able to continue their normal activities.

Three long-term side effects that often concern patients bear special mention. Patients are often concerned about short-term memory loss or cognitive changes following radiation therapy. Again, the volume of brain irradiated, the areas of the brain irradiated, the total dose received, and the age of the patient are factors that impact the cognitive changes that are observed at least one year after treatment. The use of chemotherapy during radiation may also be associated with cognitive changes. Although the best studies of the effects of whole brain radiation therapy on cognition, as measured by IQ testing, have been done in children, there is ample evidence to suggest that adults can suffer cognitive loss, particularly in short-term memory, following whole brain radiation therapy. Although partial brain irradiation has also shown some effect on cognition, the effects tend to be less pronounced and may take longer to become apparent.

A second long-term side effect that may affect patients who have received relatively high-dose radiation therapy is radiation necrosis. Radiation necrosis is an area of injured normal glial cells and blood vessels. It can occur anywhere from several months to 2 to 3 years after radiation therapy. The appearance of radiation necrosis on CT or MRI may be indistinguishable from tumor recurrence. There is typically an area of enhancement, surrounded by edema, and the area may appear to enlarge over subsequent scans. Patients experiencing radiation necrosis may develop neurological symptoms such as weakness, loss of coordination, or visual disturbances that may mimic tumor recurrence. Surgery may be required to remove the area of necrosis. Radiation necrosis is more common after high doses of focused radiation therapy, such as radiosurgery or brachytherapy.

A third complication of radiation therapy, although rare, may occur several years after treatment. A secondary malignancy is a cancer that develops as a result of previous cancer therapy. Secondary malignancies may occur in patients who have received curative radiation therapy for childhood or early adult brain tumors, or may occur following whole brain radiation therapy for acute leukemia. The original tumor has not recurred, but a new type of tumor—often a malignant glioma—appears within the radiation field. The risk of secondary malignant tumors 15 years after radiation therapy is estimated at less than 5%. However, a secondary malignant tumor may be more difficult to treat, since the patient has previously had radiation therapy to the same area. In addition to secondary malignancies, benign tumors, including meningiomas and nerve sheath tumors, may also develop following radiation therapy.

Radiation Therapy

M.L.'s comment:

The side effects that I experienced during radiation were primarily fatigue and hair loss. Some days the fatigue was greater than others, but I soon realized that I needed to just give in to the fact that I was tired and needed to take a nap. However, a nap or a good night's sleep may not always relieve your fatigue. It's very common for cancer patients to experience fatigue, and it can affect you in many ways other than just feeling tired or weary. In addition to not having as much energy during the day, I experienced periods of depression. I would begin to cry whenever I would talk to a loved one—especially my mother or sister. Because they both live far away, I felt sort of alone. I really wasn't alone, though. In fact, I had an overwhelming amount of support and comfort throughout the worst part of my treatments. Despite such support, I found that I couldn't help crying at times. In my case, this aspect of fatigue didn't go on for too long.

If you find that you're having a difficult time with fatigue, you should know that there are things that you can do to minimize the feelings of fatigue and frustration. Try to remember to rest when you feel like you need it; don't fight the fatigue. Also, try to eat right. Eat foods that will give you energy. Your doctors should be able to give you some helpful ideas of what you should and shouldn't eat. Try to get some sort of exercise every day, even if it's just a short walk around the block. I found that just getting outside and getting a bit of fresh air every day helped to relieve some of the fatigue that I was feeling. And finally, don't forget to have some sort of a social life. Just because you have a brain tumor doesn't mean you have to stop having fun. A reduction in your social life will help to conserve some of your energy, but you shouldn't feel like you have to cut out all of the things that you enjoy doing. It's all about being able to prioritize and balance the activities you have to do in order to keep from being too tired for activities that you love to do.

35. My tumor was completely resected, but I understand that there could still be microscopic tumor left behind. How does the radiation oncologist decide how much of the brain to radiate if nothing is visible on the MRI?

The MRI scans performed before surgery help determine how much area around the tumor cavity should be included in the radiation field. For tumors that infiltrate into the surrounding brain, a margin of at least 2 centimeters around the tumor is often recommended. Well-circumscribed tumors may require a smaller margin, and tumors with extensive surrounding edema may require a larger margin. Clinical trials that include radiation therapy often specify how the radiation field will be designed and the margin that will be used.

36. A patient in my support group said that he had whole brain radiation therapy. My radiation oncologist said that whole brain radiation isn't appropriate for my tumor. Why do some patients have whole brain radiation and

others do not? Are there more side effects from whole brain radiation?

Studies of patients with malignant gliomas who received whole brain radiation therapy showed that tumor recurrence frequently occurred within 2 to 5 centimeters of the original site. Those studies also found that new tumors separate and distant from the original tumor occurred in only about 5% of patients. Therefore, most radiation for malignant glioma (and many other solitary brain tumors) is limited to the area of the tumor and a margin around the tumor.

Whole brain radiation is still recommended for some tumors that are more likely to spread throughout the brain. Tumors that have metastasized from a systemic cancer such as breast or lung cancer are usually treated with whole brain radiation. Some primary tumors with multiple sites of disease at diagnosis (such as lymphoma, germinoma, and gliomatosis cerebri) may also be treated with whole brain radiation therapy.

Whole brain radiation therapy may be associated with an increased risk of narrowing of the blood vessels of the brain, radiation necrosis, and memory impairment. For this reason, whole brain radiation therapy is often less that radiation limited to a solitary focus of tumor (4000 cGy vs. 6000 cGy).

37. What is the difference between stereotactic radiosurgery (SRS) and Gamma Knife? Which patients should

receive SRS and which should receive Gamma Knife?

Stereotactic radiosurgery (SRS) and Gamma Knife are both forms of highly focused radiation therapy. Despite the names, neither involves surgery. Both procedures are performed by a team of neurosurgeons, radiation oncologists, and radiation physicists. Some communities have both a Gamma Knife unit and a linear accelerator that is modified for SRS.

Stereotactic radiosurgery can be performed by a linear accelerator modified to produce a focused beam of photons to a small (3 to 4 cm) tumor. The fixation of the patient's head in a stereotactic frame enables the radiation source to move around the target over a period of minutes, delivering a single high dose. Computer imaging can direct the beam to conform to the shape of the tumor. With some types of fixation systems, the dose can also be fractionated over several treatments.

Gamma Knife uses cobalt as a radiation source. The radiation sources are symmetrically arranged in a helmet-like pattern over the patient's head. The radiation beams converge on the target with a high degree of accuracy, but the radiation sources do not move. Gamma Knife is not fractionated, but multiple lesions can be treated in the same setting, if necessary.

Both SRS and Gamma Knife are best suited for small, spherical tumors, particularly metastases and acoustic neuromas. Gamma Knife is also used to treat vascular malformations and other non-tumor conditions in the brain. While it is difficult to compare Gamma Knife outcomes and SRS outcomes, the Gamma Knife procedure appears to provide more tumor control and have fewer complications. However, the modifications to the linear accelerator used for SRS may also be used for the treatment of other types of tumors, meaning facilities that use this procedure can treat a variety of conditions, whereas Gamma Knife facilities only treat intracranial lesions.

Most patients will have access to a center with Gamma Knife or SRS. Your doctor may prefer one type of treatment over the other for your specific type of tumor. More information regarding Gamma Knife or SRS treatment will be available at your initial evaluation with your radiation oncologist.

38. I have seen two radiation oncologists. One says that he uses three-dimensional imaging to plan treatment. He says this targets the tumor more precisely, which makes the treatment safer. The other radiation oncologist says that the precision of three-dimensional imaging does not make the treatment safer; only the total dose of radiation determines the extent of side effects. Who's right?

Both doctors are right. When a patient undergoes radiation therapy, the total dose of radiation delivered must not exceed safe parameters, and radiation delivery must avoid those sensitive brain structures that are not affected by the tumor. **Conformal radiation therapy,** a three-dimensional radiation treatment, uses images from CT or MRI to plan precise fields of radiation that can be contoured around sensitive structures such as the eyes or the brainstem. By using conformal radiation therapy, the total radiation dose delivered to the tumor may be the same as conventional external beam radiation therapy, but the dose delivered to the surrounding normal brain may be less (Color Plate 6).

The dose delivered to the tumor and the dose delivered to the surrounding brain may cause side effects. Doses of radiation therapy high enough to cause tumor necrosis can create a focus of dead tissue that may eventually cause symptoms. If this occurs, the dead tissue may need to be surgically removed. It may seem optimal to simply limit the dose of radiation to the normal brain surrounding the tumor, but some tumors spread into the normal brain far away from the tumor mass that appears on an MRI. Treating this area of normal brain with a lower dose of radiation may place the patient at risk for tumor recurrence, and a subsequent course of radiation therapy may not be possible if there is an overlap with the previous radiation field.

39. What is interstitial brachytherapy?

Interstitial brachytherapy (interstitial = within space, brachy = short) refers to radiation therapy that is administered from the inside of the tumor cavity. Sources of radiation include iodine or iridium. In this treatment approach, radioactive seeds or pellets

Conformal radiation therapy

therapy that uses images from CT and MRI to plan precise fields of radiation that may be contoured around structures such as the eyes or the brainstem.

Radiation Therapy

are implanted directly into the tumor cavity. The seeds or pellets deliver a low dose of radiation continuously to nearby surrounding tissue. Patients who are suitable candidates for brachytherapy have a well-circumscribed, resectable tumor less than 5 centimeters in diameter.

Recently, a balloon catheter system called GliaSite was developed for placement into a tumor resection cavity. The balloon is inflated to a diameter of 2 to 4 centimeters and filled with a radioactive iodine solution, Iotrex. The solution remains in place for 3 to 6 days. Then the Iotrex and balloon catheter are removed.

Although in some studies brachytherapy has been associated with an improvement in overall survival, some patients have needed another operation to remove radiation necrosis. In the initial GliaSite study, no patients required another operation for radiation necrosis, and the median survival time for patients who underwent the procedure exceeded one year.

40. I had a biopsy of a tumor in my left hemisphere that measures 2 × 2 centimeters. The biopsy determined the tumor was a low-grade astrocytoma. I have seen a radiation oncologist who suggested immediate radiation therapy. When I got a second opinion from another radiation oncologist, he suggested that radiation therapy could be

delayed for a few years. Why are the recommendations so different?

Treatment recommendations for brain tumors, particularly for low-grade gliomas, are guided by many factors. To help guide treatment decisions, many doctors refer to practice guidelines. The National Comprehensive Cancer Network (NCCN), a committee composed of neuro-oncologists, radiation oncologists, and neurosurgeons around the country, publishes such practice guidelines. The NCCN practice guidelines provide treatment recommendations that are based on current cancer research as well as the clinical experience of the committee members.

Many physicians use the NCCN guidelines as a reference, but many do not. Some academic centers and research institutions have developed their own guidelines for the treatment of specific brain tumors. However, all practice guidelines assume that doctors exercise good medical judgment in the patient's care, taking into consideration the patient's age and general health. Even the NCCN recommendations are not a "cookbook" approach for the treatment of any type of brain tumor. This is why different doctors may have different recommendations for treatment. Practice guidelines provide doctors with information that helps guide treatment, but the factors involved in your specific case also impact treatment decisions.

Low-grade gliomas can be quite variable in their behavior, making general recommendations difficult. Some gliomas are surgically resectable, but others spread into the surrounding brain and cannot be removed safely. If the tumor can be completely resected, some studies have shown that survival improves. Other studies have demonstrated that aggressive surgical resection does not improve survival.

Radiation therapy is often recommended for patients with low-grade gliomas that cannot be resected. However, because some patients have few, if any, symptoms, their doctors may recommend delaying radiation therapy until symptoms develop or until there is a change in the appearance of the tumor on MRI scan. Again, clinical trials have shown conflicting results on which approach (immediate or delayed radiation) makes a difference in overall survival.

At least 50% of low-grade tumors do become more malignant over a period of several years, progressing to anaplastic astrocytoma (Grade 3) or glioblastoma multiforme (Grade 4). This change can occur whether or not the patient has received radiation therapy. However, patients who have previously received a full course of radiation therapy may not be able to receive more radiation if the tumor recurs as a higher grade tumor. Also, radiation can increase the risk of developing a second tumor, but this risk is considered very small (probably less than 5% fifteen years after radiation).

Although neither group of physicians you have seen recommended chemotherapy, some clinical trials have studied regimens such as PCV (Procarbazine, CCNU, and Vincristine) or Temodar in low-grade glioma patients with or without radiation therapy. It is not yet clear how chemotherapy impacts on overall survival. Particularly for patients who have a low-grade oligodendroglioma, or who have mixed oligo-astrocytoma, chemotherapy may allow patients to defer radiation therapy for months or years.

In summary, despite the development of practice guidelines, it is still up to you and your doctor when you should undergo radiation therapy. You may also want to consider participation in a clinical trial studying new treatment approaches to the management of low-grade glioma.

41. Losing part of my hair during radiation therapy has been very hard for me. What can I do to make the experience more tolerable?

Hair loss in the area that received radiation is very common during radiation therapy. Hair loss from chemotherapy, on the other hand, affects hair all over the body. Being prepared for the loss of your hair will make the experience somewhat easier. Even before radiation or chemotherapy begins, many people look for a wig or hairpiece in the same color or style as their natural hair to ease the transition to hair loss. Your doctor may write a prescription for a wig or hairpiece because the loss of your hair is associated with your cancer treatment.

Cutting your hair short before you begin to lose it makes it somewhat more manageable when it does begin to fall out. You can also use a mild shampoo and conditioner and avoid blow-drying it to help avoid irritating your scalp.

Scarves, turbans, hats, and other head coverings can be used on the days when you prefer not to wear a hair-

piece. The American Cancer Society publishes a cata-
logue of wigs and various head coverings. Also, many
communities have a boutique designed for men and
women who have hair loss related to cancer treatment.

M.L.'s comment:

*Although the amount of hair loss that people have after
radiation is variable, more than likely you'll lose at least
some of it. I did, and it was very upsetting to see those
first clumps of hair come out in the bathroom sink. I
knew it would happen; I just didn't know when it
would happen. I tried to prepare for it, but I still cried
when it happened. You have to keep telling yourself it's
all part of the healing process. I continued to remind
myself that the radiation that was making my hair fall
out was also continuing to eat away at those "bad cells"
in my brain, and that was a good thing. I just tried to
stay strong through all of it. I kept telling myself that my
hair would grow back. I found that wearing a "doo rag"
on my head with a baseball cap over it made me feel
kind of cool. My husband has a motorcycle and he took
me to a shop where they sold motorcycles, clothing, and
accessories. One of the accessories that motocyclists wear
when they are riding is a "doo rag." It keeps the rider's
hair from flying all over the place, and it makes the hel-
met a bit more comfortable. I found that they looked a lot
better than a scarf or bandanna, so I started wearing
them every day. It was funny when people started asking
me where I had bought them.*

What to Expect during Radiation Therapy

Patients who will receive radiation therapy as part of
their treatment for a primary or metastatic brain tumor
meet with a radiation oncologist, a doctor who special-

izes in treating tumors with radiation therapy. Although a radiation oncologist may visit with you following surgery while you are still in the hospital, most radiation therapy is conducted on an outpatient basis.

After discussing the potential benefits and risks of radiation therapy, the radiation oncologist discusses the detailed treatment plan and the patient signs an **informed consent**. This explains potential risks and complications of the treatment.

The patient's MRI or CT scans are reviewed by the radiation oncologist to determine the **target volume** (the area that will be irradiated). Sometimes, additional microscopic tumor cells grow at the edge of the tumor visualized on brain scans. The radiation oncologist takes this into account by including a margin of 1 to 3 centimeters around the tumor in the target volume. The radiation oncologist also notes sensitive areas that should not receive full doses of radiation, such as the eyes or the brain stem.

The radiation oncologist and the **radiation physicist** determine the doses of radiation that the patient will receive. They calculate the total amount of radiation to the tumor as well as the amount that will be distributed over the remaining portions of the brain. With conventional radiation therapy, areas adjacent to the tumor may receive a percentage of the total dose (Color Plate 6).

To make sure that the patient receives the dose in exactly the same configuration day after day, the radiation technicians create a custom "mask" that holds the patient in place. This is often a netlike device that

Radiation Therapy

Informed Consent

process of explaining to the patient all risks and complications of a procedure or treatment before it is done. Informed consents are signed by the patient, a parent of a minor child, or a legal representative.

Target volume

the three-dimensional portion of an organ or organs, identified from the patient's scans or x rays, to receive radiation therapy treatments.

allows the patient to breathe normally but still holds the head firmly in place during treatment.

With the patient in position, x rays may be taken to provide a **simulation** of the exact treatment field. When the radiation oncologist is satisfied with the treatment planning, the actual treatment begins. The treatment session, once planning is completed, is typically brief, often lasting about 15 minutes.

During treatment, the linear accelerator, a source of radiation therapy, rotates around the patient very precisely. Different angles may be used, from the sides of the head or front to back, to focus intersecting beams of radiation at the tumor. The treatment may be modified during radiation therapy if a smaller section of the tumor will receive a "boost." This may require more CT or MRI planning and a second planning session.

Typically the radiation oncologist sees the patient at least weekly during treatment. The radiation oncologist may recommend treatment with steroids if the patient develops symptoms of swelling around the tumor during radiation therapy. Any other side effects of treatment are also discussed with the radiation oncologist.

After completing radiation therapy, the radiation oncologist reviews the post-treatment MRI with the patient. Because of changes in the tumor and surrounding tissue that may occur during radiation therapy, the MRI is usually evaluated several weeks after radiation therapy ends. However, the tumor may continue to shrink for several months after the completion of radiation therapy, so additional scans are often recommended to assess the success of treatment.

PART SIX

Chemotherapy and Other Drug Therapy

What is the blood-brain barrier, and how does it determine which drugs are used in brain tumor treatment?

What is chemotherapy?

What are the most common drugs used to treat brain tumors? What are their side effects?

More . . .

42. What is the blood-brain barrier? How does it determine which drugs are used in brain tumor treatment?

The tiny blood vessels or capillaries of the brain that deliver oxygen and nutrients to the cells differ from the capillaries of other organs. The walls of the capillaries of most of the body are porous so that molecules move freely from the bloodstream into the tissues. The walls of the capillaries of the brain, on the other hand, are more tightly joined together. This tight seam or "junction" restricts the movement of larger molecules, including drug molecules, into the brain. The blood-brain barrier refers to the limitation imposed on drugs and other substances from crossing the capillary walls into brain tissues.

Clearly, there are many drugs that readily pass into the brain (for example, alcohol, cocaine, and all types of "recreational" drugs!), but other drugs have physical characteristics that prevent their passage through the capillaries. Some brain tumors have more "leaky" capillaries, and therefore do not have an intact blood-brain barrier. These tumors tend to show an area of bright contrast enhancement on MRI when intravenous gadolinium has been used (see Question 16).

Some chemotherapy drugs, including carmustine (BCNU), lomustine (CCNU), temozolomide (Temodar), and procarbazine (Matulane), have the ability to cross the intact blood-brain barrier. The drugs cisplatin and carboplatin do not cross the intact blood-brain barrier well, but they may be effective in malignant tumors, which have capillaries that are more porous.

The significance of the blood-brain barrier in determining the success of chemotherapy in brain tumors has been debated for many years. The presence of "leaky" capillaries within the tumor may allow the chemotherapy drug to kill more of the surrounding tumor cells. It is possible to open the blood-brain barrier temporarily with other drugs. This process, called blood-brain barrier disruption, has been developed in some research centers as a way to achieve higher concentrations of chemotherapy to the tumor and to the surrounding brain tissues, which may contain scattered tumor cells. This has been particularly useful in treating primary CNS lymphoma, which is a very chemotherapy-sensitive tumor.

Unfortunately, the blood-brain barrier does not prevent systemic cancers, such as breast cancer and lung cancer, from spreading into the brain and spinal fluid. It may, however, limit the penetration of chemotherapy drugs into the brain. For example, a lung cancer patient taking chemotherapy may have shrinkage of his lung cancer at the same time that metastases in the brain are continuing to grow.

43. What is chemotherapy? What are the most common drugs used to treat brain tumors? What are their side effects?

Chemotherapy refers to the medication used to treat cancer that has direct effects on the growth and proliferation of cancer cells. There are hundreds of chemotherapy drugs, and they are divided into different classes depending on how they affect the cell. Most chemotherapy drugs interfere with the reproductive cycle of cancer cells by affecting their DNA, but

Chemotherapy
the use of chemical agents (drugs) to treat cancer.

some block other steps in cell division. Unfortunately, the effects of chemotherapy on some of the body's normal cells, particularly the rapidly dividing cells of the bone marrow, can cause considerable toxicity. Because the bone marrow produces red blood cells, white blood cells, and platelets, chemotherapy can kill these cells, sometimes placing the patient at risk for infection or bleeding.

Chemotherapy is usually given in **cycles.** Each cycle consists of the day or days in which chemotherapy is given and the time it takes for bone marrow to recover or other toxicity to resolve. The cycle length varies according to the drug or combination of drugs; it may be as short as 3 weeks or as long as 8 weeks.

It is difficult to list all of the drugs that have been used in the treatment of primary and metastatic tumors. However, some drugs have been developed specifically for the treatment of primary brain tumors. Others have shown effectiveness in clinical trials; some of these drugs are already approved by the **Food and Drug Administration (FDA)** to treat other conditions. These drugs may be considered **off-label** for use in the treatment of brain tumors (see Question 60). Some drugs are best known by their generic name and others by their trade name; the names used most commonly will be used for simplicity.

Food and Drug Administration (FDA)

a federal institution charged with approving and regulating medications, foods, and other products for human consumption.

Off-label drug

a drug that is approved by the FDA for one type of treatment but may be prescribed for other conditions.

The drugs BCNU (carmustine) and CCNU (lomustine) are some of the oldest drugs used to treat astrocytomas, oligodendrogliomas, and many other types of brain tumors. BCNU is an intravenous drug; and its chemically related cousin, CCNU, is an oral drug.

BCNU and CCNU have good penetration across the blood-brain barrier, but they may affect blood cell counts for several weeks; therefore, these drugs are commonly given in cycles 6 to 8 weeks apart. In addition to their effects on blood cell counts, these drugs can cause lung scarring (pulmonary fibrosis), a condition that may cause shortness of breath. BCNU and CCNU have been used in combination with other chemotherapy drugs. For example, CCNU is commonly used in combination with procarbazine and vincristine in a drug regimen known as PCV.

BCNU has been incorporated into a wafer, which is designed to dissolve in the brain when placed into the surgical cavity following tumor resection. The Gliadel wafer does not affect blood cell counts or cause lung toxicity, but it may not be used in patients whose tumors cannot be resected. When using Gliadel, the neurosurgeon must take precautions to make sure spinal fluid containing BCNU does not contaminate the surgical wound. Currently, Gliadel is approved to treat glioblastoma multiforme, although off-label use of the wafer has included patients with other resectable primary or metastatic tumors.

Temozolomide (Temodar) is an oral drug developed in Europe that was approved for treatment of recurrent anaplastic astrocytoma in the United States in 1999. Since that time, many other tumor types have been studied in clinical trials with Temodar. Some clinical trials have explored the use of Temodar in combination with other drugs and with radiation therapy. Many different administration schedules have also been used, but the most common schedule used in the United

States recommends that Temodar be taken daily, at bed-time, for 5 days, every 4 weeks. Most patients tolerate Temodar well without experiencing significant effects on blood counts. Temodar has not been shown to cause lung damage. It may cause nausea and constipation, but both can usually be controlled with other medications.

Procarbazine (Matulane) is an oral chemotherapy drug that may be used alone or in combination with other chemotherapy drugs. This drug, however, interacts with other drugs, including antihistamines, narcotics, some nausea medications, and alcohol. Procarbazine can also cause high blood pressure when used in combination with foods high in tyramine, such as brewer's yeast, chicken livers, bananas, and aged cheese. A study comparing Temodar and procarbazine in recurrent glioblastoma found that Temodar causes less toxicity and appears to be more effective than procarbazine, although procarbazine is still widely used in combination therapy.

Methotrexate has been used primarily to treat CNS lymphoma. It is often given in high doses and followed with administration of leucovorin, a drug that acts as an antidote for methotrexate toxicity in normal cells. High doses are necessary to penetrate into spinal fluid and treat leptomeningeal cancer cells.

Carboplatin (Paraplatin) and cisplatin are commonly used to treat lung cancer, ovarian cancer, and other malignancies. They have been used intravenously and intra-arterially in primary brain tumors. Both are commonly given with other drugs. Cisplatin may cause kidney damage, peripheral neuropathy (numbness and tingling, particularly in the lower extremities), and severe nausea.

Cyclophosphamide (**Cytoxan**) is an intravenous drug that has been used for pediatric and adult brain tumors such as medulloblastoma. It causes low blood cell counts and nausea.

CPT–11 (Camptosar, also called irinotecan) is an intravenous drug that was originally approved to treat colon cancer. Clinical trials have shown that CPT–11 is effective in treating malignant glioma. Several different doses and schedules have been used.

Etoposide (VP–16) has been used orally and intravenously to treat many different types of cancer. It has been used in combination with other drugs to treat medulloblastoma, germinoma, and primitive neuroectodermal tumors. It has also been used to treat metastatic small cell lung cancer.

Vincristine (Oncovin) is rarely used as a single drug in the treatment of cancer, but it is often used in combination with other drugs because it does not affect blood cell counts. However, vincristine may cause numbness, weakness, constipation, impotence, and other significant side effects. This drug is given intravenously.

Many other chemotherapy drugs have been used alone or in combination with other drugs to treat primary and metastatic brain tumors. Your oncologist or oncology nurse will give you references and information regarding the possible side effects of the drugs recommended to you before you start treatment.

44. Why are my blood cell counts affected by chemotherapy? Are low blood cell counts dangerous? What can I do to keep my blood cell counts high during chemotherapy?

Because many chemotherapy drugs interfere with cell division, the rapidly dividing cells of the bone marrow—the white cells, red cells, and platelets—are the "innocent bystanders" of the toxic effects of chemotherapy. Fortunately, blood cell counts usually recover rapidly, often within days, but some drugs have longer effects on the blood cell counts. Your doctor or nurse will explain to you which of your blood cell counts may be affected by your chemotherapy and what you should expect while your blood cell counts may be low. If your blood cell counts remain lower than expected, it may become necessary for your doctor to reduce the dosage of your chemotherapy.

White blood cells (**neutrophils**, **lymphocytes**, and **monocytes**) protect your body against infection. Neutrophils, also called segmented neutrophils or polymorphonuclear leukocytes, are the first line of defense against bacterial infections and fungal infections. These cells often multiply rapidly during the early stages of an infection. For example, a high white blood cell count may signal a serious infection such as pneumonia. However, if the patient is undergoing chemotherapy, the white blood cell count may be lower than usual. Particularly when the neutrophil

Neutrophil
type of white blood cell.

Lymphocytes
type of white blood cell found in lymphatic tissue such as lymph nodes, spleen, and bone marrow.

Monocytes
type of white blood cell normally found in lymph nodes, spleen, bone marrow and within tissue.

count is very low (a condition called **neutropenia**), the patient is at more risk for severe infection. It is important to notify your doctor if you develop a fever, cough, or other symptoms of infection when your white cell count may be low. A number of different drugs, including sargramostim (Leukine), filgrastim (Neupogen), and pegfilgrastim (Neulasta), may be administered by injection to stimulate recovery of your neutrophil count to normal. In some situations, your doctor may need to hospitalize you to treat fever or infection while your white blood cell count is low.

The red blood cell count may also be affected by chemotherapy. A low red blood cell count (**anemia**) may result from a number of other causes, including iron deficiency. For this reason, you should be careful to include iron-rich foods in your diet while you are on chemotherapy. Anemia can cause fatigue and shortness of breath. In severe cases of anemia, it may be necessary to have a transfusion of red blood cells. Epoetin alfa (Procrit), an injectable red blood cell growth factor, may be recommended by your oncologist if your red blood cell count falls during chemotherapy.

Platelets are important in normal clotting, and a very low platelet count (**thrombocytopenia**) may be associated with severe bleeding. If necessary, a low platelet count can be treated with transfusion. Oprevelkin (Neumega) is an injectable drug that is used to stimulate the recovery of platelets. It is administered for several days following chemotherapy, when thrombocytopenia is anticipated.

45. I've heard terrible things about chemotherapy and the nausea and

Neutropenia
a lower than normal neutrophil count.

Thrombocytopenia
low platelet count.

Chemotherapy and Other Drug Therapy

vomiting associated with it. Will I be very ill while I'm on chemotherapy?

Fortunately, many of the side effects of chemotherapy that were distressing to patients in the past are now avoided because of widespread use of **antiemetic** (antinausea) medications that were developed specifically for chemotherapy. Medications such as ondansetron (Zofran), granisetron (Kytril), and dolesetron (Anzemet) can be given intravenously or orally before chemotherapy. These drugs, unlike some of the older medications, do not cause sedation, making it safer for patients to receive chemotherapy in the outpatient setting. Many of the chemotherapy drugs used to treat brain tumors, such as BCNU, CCNU, and Temodar, may cause nausea. Oncologists recommend that patients receive antiemetic medication *before* taking the chemotherapy rather than waiting to see if nausea will develop. It is particularly important to prevent vomiting when taking an oral chemotherapy drug, because it cannot be "doubled up" if a dose is missed.

Antiemetics
drugs that prevent nausea and vomiting.

M.L.'s comment:

I think the fear of nausea and vomiting is the most common concern with chemotherapy. It certainly was for me! I rarely experienced any sickness while I was on chemotherapy and I could hardly believe it. I took Temodar for 23 months and only had severe nausea on the first night that I took it. I think I probably was so nervous about whether or not I would get sick that I probably brought the nausea and vomiting on myself. I'll never really know whether it was the drug or my nerves that made me sick, but I do know that I took the antinausea medication every single time that I took my Temodar and it helped.

The side effect that I DID have was just a general feeling of being tired, but not so tired that I couldn't go to work. There were days that I would go home early or go in late. For the first couple of days that I was on chemotherapy, I was fine. I didn't feel tired at all. However, as the week went on and more chemotherapy was in my body, I started to become more tired. I remember wanting to sleep in later than usual, and I would fall asleep earlier in the evening than usual. This wasn't really a bad thing. I just felt like it was the reality of being on chemo, and hey, it was a lot better than feeling nauseous.

Another side effect that I felt was loss of appetite. For me, that was a good thing because I had gained so much weight while I was on steroids that I wanted to lose some weight. In talking with others who were on Temodar, I found that the loss of appetite affects everyone differently. There were some people who said they didn't have much of an appetite for anything. Others, like me, only had a slight loss of appetite. The good news was that my normal appetite came back shortly after I finished each round of chemotherapy.

One other side effect that occurred while I was taking Temodar was constipation. If you've ever been really constipated you know that it isn't something that you want to experience very often. I found that I didn't experience the constipation if I took a powdered laxative mixed in with orange juice once a day for every day that I was on chemotherapy. Most of the time, I would extend taking the laxative a few more days until I felt like the chemotherapy had gone through my system and my appetite was back to normal.

All in all, my experience with Temodar was surprisingly positive. I didn't get sick and I didn't lose my hair. Yes, I was a little fatigued and my appetite was down, but this only lasted for about 5 to 7 days. Once I figured out how to address the constipation that wasn't even an issue any more. In short, I'll take the fatigue, loss of appetite, and the constipation over NOT getting sick or losing my hair any day of the week!

46. I have seen two oncologists who have recommended chemotherapy for my tumor, but one said that I should take it immediately after radiation therapy and the other said I should take it when the tumor grows or becomes more symptomatic. Who's right? Does it make any difference in the outcome?

The decision of *when* to take chemotherapy is only one part of the problem. The other issues are *what* chemotherapy to take, *how long* to take it, and *why* chemotherapy should be taken for the particular type of tumor you have.

As with other issues regarding treatment, if you are considering participation in a clinical trial, you must make certain that you will keep your eligibility for the trial. Some clinical trials do not allow patients who have had chemotherapy to participate. Others will not allow patients to participate after radiation therapy until their tumor grows enough to become apparent on MRI. If participating in a specific clinical trial is important to you, be sure to contact the center offering the trial before you begin another treatment.

In general, chemotherapy is offered to patients who have a high likelihood of recurrence, either because the tumor cannot be cured by surgery or radiation therapy alone, or because a previous randomized trial indicated that the addition of chemotherapy prolonged survival. For low-grade glioma, for example, a long duration of survival is common following treatment with radiation therapy, but only a few trials have been completed using chemotherapy immediately after radiation therapy. In one of these trials, CCNU offered no improvement in survival for patients with low-grade gliomas over radiation therapy alone. On the other hand, in patients with high-grade gliomas, the addition of BCNU or CCNU to radiation therapy appeared to improve survival. The initial studies of Temodar were conducted in patients who had had regrowth of tumor weeks or months after radiation therapy. More recent studies of using Temodar immediately following radiation therapy in patients with high-grade gliomas have also suggested an improvement in survival. Other studies have combined radiation therapy and Temodar in newly diagnosed patients. It is not yet clear which approach results in the best overall survival.

Theoretically, the optimal time to begin chemotherapy for any type of cancer is when there are only a few tumor cells present. If surgery and radiation therapy have eliminated the majority of tumor cells, the few that remain may be treated with chemotherapy successfully. However, this scenario is only true when the chemotherapy chosen is known to be effective against the tumor cells. Because of the differences in their sensitivity to chemotherapy, it is anticipated that some cells will remain after treatment with a given chemotherapy agent. This is why multiple drugs have been used either simultaneously or sequentially to treat residual tumor.

For most brain tumors, the optimal duration of chemotherapy treatment that follows surgery and radiation therapy is not known. In the past, when drugs such as CCNU and BCNU were the mainstay of treatment, few patients could tolerate several months of therapy because of the development of toxicity to the bone marrow and lungs. Newer drugs such as Temodar are not as toxic, and many patients can tolerate treatment for a year or longer. However, if there is no evidence of residual tumor on MRI after several months of treatment, it is still not clear whether patients should continue chemotherapy or continue follow-up without active treatment (see Question 52).

Remember that there is not just one right answer to questions regarding treatment. A number of different treatment approaches have been developed over the past ten years, and recommendations continue to evolve from the results of clinical trials. If you desire aggressive treatment because of the possibility of residual tumor, you should communicate this to your oncologist.

47. Why are some drugs given orally, through a vein, or through an artery, whereas other drugs are delivered into the spinal fluid or into the tumor cavity?

All of the drugs commonly used in the treatment of cancer have been studied for several years in research animals and in clinical trials. During those studies, some drugs were noted to be easily absorbed through the gastrointestinal tract when taken orally, a characteristic called **bioavailability.** However, some drugs are not absorbed or lose their effectiveness when administered orally. These drugs have not been manufactured in an oral form and are only available as an injectable (usually intravenous) preparation. Temodar is an oral drug with good bioavailability; CPT–11 has poor bioavailability and is always given intravenously.

Bioavailability

chemical property of a drug describing its absorption through the gastrointestinal tract when taken orally.

Relatively few drugs have been studied by directly injecting them into an artery that supplies the tumor (intra-arterial administration). Also, only a few drugs have been proven safe to inject directly into spinal fluid (intrathecal administration). In general, research centers that specialize in drug development use animal models to determine the safety and effectiveness of drugs to use by these special routes. The chemotherapy wafer Gliadel, which contains the drug BCNU, is currently the only chemotherapy approved for administration into the tumor cavity (intracavitary administration). Methotrexate is one of the few drugs that can be given intravenously, intra-arterially, intrathecally, and orally.

48. I have had surgery, radiation therapy, and chemotherapy. My oncologist recently said that after a year of treatment I have had a "complete remission." I asked him if this is the same as being cured, but he said no. What is the difference between remission and cure?

Remission (from the Latin word *remissio*, to send back) means that the symptoms of a disease and the objective evidence of the disease have partially or completely resolved. A **partial remission (PR)** means that

Partial remission (PR)

shrinkage or partial disappearance of tumor, but with evidence that some of the tumor still exists.

some evidence of the tumor remains. In a clinical trial, at least a 50% reduction in the original size of the tumor must occur before a patient is considered a PR. The complete resolution of *all* signs and symptoms of disease is a **complete remission (CR).** Because of the post-treatment abnormalities that may persist for several months on MRI, it can be difficult to define when a brain tumor patient achieves CR.

Complete remission (CR)

the complete resolution of all signs and symptoms of disease.

However, having a normal MRI scan for months or years does not necessarily mean that a patient is cured. Most people would define cure as the *permanent* eradication of disease. It would be impossible to verify over a period as short as 12 months that the disease is permanently eradicated. In the absence of effective treatment, microscopic disease may eventually grow back into visible tumor.

Although most patients want to know what their chances are for cure, the answer is never 100%, and it is never 0%. The chance of achieving remission, however, may be quite high. The next question typically asked is: "How long will the remission last?" Because of the variation in growth rates among different types of brain tumors, this can also vary widely. For example, primary CNS lymphoma is a malignant tumor that may involve the brain and spinal fluid. If a patient completes treatment and the MRI of the brain shows no evidence of disease, but the patient still has malignant cells in the spinal fluid, the patient's "response" to treatment would be considered a PR. A patient is considered a CR only when *all* evidence of disease has resolved with treatment. In some studies, the proportion of CNS lymphoma patients achieving a complete remission may exceed 50%. Some of those patients may be cured.

However, because of the known risk of relapse, these patients are followed regularly for any recurrence of disease. In fact, a complete remission may last only a matter of weeks after discontinuing treatment.

It is important to understand that in using the word "remission," your doctor is not trying to avoid the word "cure." Your doctor is merely trying to describe as accurately as possible the presence or absence of disease.

49. My cancer was found in the spinal fluid. My doctor says that chemotherapy can be given directly into the spinal fluid with an Ommaya reservoir. What is an Ommaya reservoir and how is it used for chemotherapy?

For patients who have cancer cells in the spinal fluid, or **leptomeningeal spread**, small doses of chemotherapy can be injected into the spinal fluid to circulate in the ventricles and over and around the spinal cord and spinal nerves. Although some patients receive chemotherapy injections with a spinal tap or lumbar puncture, this may be impractical or technically difficult for patients who require treatment for several months.

An **Ommaya reservoir** is a hollow, slightly dome-shaped, silicone device that is attached to a catheter, surgically implanted by a neurosurgeon in the operating room. The catheter is threaded though a small hole in the skull, into the nondominant cerebral hemisphere, often the right frontal lobe (Figure 4). The

Leptomeningeal spread

the spread of cancer cells through the spinal fluid, producing a coating around the brain or spinal cord.

Ommaya reservoir

a device for administering chemotherapy into the spinal fluid.

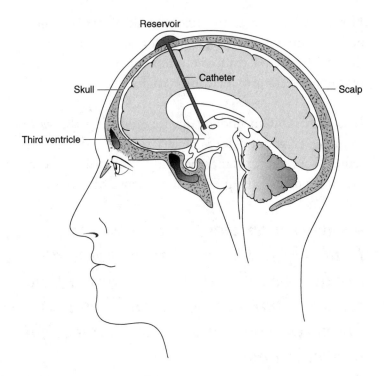

Figure 4   Ommaya reservoir.

hollow reservoir is slipped between the skin of the scalp and the skull and sutured in place. The slightly rounded surface of the reservoir allows your doctor to locate its placement, and the surface of the skin is cleansed with antibacterial solution. A butterfly needle is inserted through the skin into the dome to "access" the reservoir. Spinal fluid is removed by slowly aspirating with a syringe, and chemotherapy is then administered by injecting it into the reservoir and catheter. Most patients have no discomfort when chemotherapy is administered through the Ommaya reservoir, and the procedure can be easily performed within minutes on an outpatient basis.

Strict adherence to sterile technique is essential when the reservoir is accessed because introduction of infection into the spinal fluid can be life threatening. Fortunately, once the skin at the insertion site of the reservoir heals, no special precautions are required on the part of the patient.

Patients who have an Ommaya reservoir for chemotherapy may require lifelong re-evaluation of the spinal fluid to detect evidence of recurrence. For this reason, the Ommaya reservoir is considered a permanent device. It is not removed at the end of treatment.

Table 4 lists drugs that have been used for intrathecal therapy. Methotrexate is by far the most common drug

Table 4   Drugs used in intrathecal therapy

Drug	Types of Cancer Treated
Methotrexate	Breast cancer, lymphoma, leukemia
Cytarabine (Ara-C)	Lymphoma, leukemia
DepoCyt (liposomal encapsulated cytarabine)	Leukemia, lymphoma
Thiotepa	Lymphoma, leukemia, breast cancer
Etopophos	Lymphoma, lung cancer, germinoma, glial tumors
Topotecan	Lymphoma, small cell lung cancer, glial tumors
Dacarbazine	Melanoma

Chemotherapy and Other Drug Therapy

used in intrathecal therapy. DepoCyt, which was approved a few years ago, is specifically formulated to persist over time, so that it requires less frequent injections. Newer drugs, such as topotecan, are still being studied in clinical trials to determine which tumors respond best. Your oncologist will provide further information about the drug and potential side effects before you begin treatment.

50. Why should I have a different type of chemotherapy if the first type didn't work?

Chemotherapy drugs that belong to different classes may have different success rates. In general, it is difficult—if not impossible—to predict at diagnosis which drug is best for a given patient. Recently, Precision Therapeutics developed testing procedures to determine the most effective drugs against a patient's tumor (Figure 5). The assay requires that a portion of the live tumor removed during surgery be submitted for analysis. Although the assay takes several days, it may be possible to identify certain drugs that are more effective against the tumor. However, there is still a chance that the patient will develop intolerable side effects to the drug. For this reason, pretreatment predictive testing is not always helpful.

In some instances, a drug that is chemically distinct from the first drug used may be more effective. For example, it is known that brain tumor cells are sometimes resistant to the chemotherapy drug BCNU. Therefore, tumor cells that are resistant to BCNU may also be resistant to CCNU because the drugs are closely related. The drug CPT–11, however, is from a

ChemoFx® Assay Final Report
Page 1 of 2

Precision Therapeutics℠
Personalizing Cancer Therapy

2516 Jane Street • Pittsburgh, PA 15203 • Phone: 800.868.9236 • Fax: 800.868.9617 • www.ptilabs.com • CLIA: 39D0914551

PATIENT: JOHN DOE
Requesting Physician: Virginia Stark-Vance, MD
Copy to:

DOB:
Facility:
Copy to:

SOC. SEC. #: - -

Copy to:

PTI Accession #:
Collection Date:
Histologic Data: cns; glioblastoma multiforme

SPECIMEN INFORMATION
PTI Received Date:
Pathology #:

Report Date:
Specimen Site: brain; left temporal

TESTING INFORMATION
Single Agents Requested: 4
Combination Agents Requested: 0
Cell Proliferation Rate: slow
Wells Tested Per Concentration: 6
Comments: n/a

Single Agents Tested: 4
Combination Agents Tested: 0
Morphology: n/a

IN VITRO RESPONSE SUMMARY

Moderate to Strong*	Modest*	Slight*	None to Minimal*
Carboplatin	Carmustine		Temozolomide
	Irinotecan		

*Drug concentrations A-F are reflected herein, with clinical concentrations represented by concentrations C and D for single agents and concentrations B and E for combination agents.

These tests are not to be used independently for purposes of medical diagnosis, prognosis, or treatment, but may be used in conjunction with other recognized, standard, laboratory and diagnostic tests and procedures, and with the experience and clinical judgment of a physician. This test was developed, and its performance characteristics determined, by Precision Therapeutics, Inc. It has not been cleared or approved by the U.S. Food and Drug Administration. The FDA has determined that such clearance or approval is not necessary. This test is used for clinical purposes and should not be regarded as investigational or for research purposes. R111102

Dennis R. Burholt, Ph.D.

ChemoFx® Assay Final Report
Page 2 of 2
PATIENT: JOHN DOE

Precision Therapeutics℠
Personalizing Cancer Therapy

MODERATE TO STRONG RESPONSE*
Indicates a response to the low concentrations tested.

Carboplatin

MODEST RESPONSE*
Indicates a response to the mid-strength concentrations tested.

Carmustine

Irinotecan

NONE TO MINIMAL RESPONSE*
Indicates either no response, or a response to only the highest concentration tested.

Temozolomide

Chart Legend
CI Value
+/-1 Standard Error

*Drug concentrations A-F are reflected herein, with clinical concentrations represented by concentrations C and D for single agents and concentrations B and E for combination agents.

These tests are not to be used independently for purposes of medical diagnosis, prognosis, or treatment, but may be used in conjunction with other recognized, standard, laboratory and diagnostic tests and procedures, and with the experience and clinical judgment of a physician. This test was developed, and its performance characteristics determined, by Precision Therapeutics, Inc. It has not been cleared or approved by the U.S. Food and Drug Administration. The FDA has determined that such clearance or approval is not necessary. This test is used for clinical purposes and should not be regarded as investigational or for research purposes. R111102

Figure 5   Sample report from Precision Therapeutics showing the effectiveness of drugs used to treat fictional patient John Doe.

different class of drugs. It kills tumor cells in a different way than BCNU or CCNU, so tumor cells may not be resistant to this drug.

51. What are the other drugs besides chemotherapy that could be used to treat my tumor?

There are a number of different drugs that have been used to treat malignant brain tumors, some alone and some in combination with chemotherapy. The majority of clinical trials to determine the effectiveness of these drugs have been conducted in patients with malignant glioma, so less is known about their usefulness in the treatment of other types of brain tumors.

Accutane (13-cis-retinoic acid) is an oral drug that has been approved for the treatment of cystic acne. It is known that some malignant gliomas have an epidermal growth factor receptor (EGFR) which, when chemically blocked, prevents cell division. Accutane appears to block the EGFR receptor. Clinical trials have shown that some patients are long-term survivors when given high-dose Accutane therapy. Accutane has also been used in combination with Temodar, improving survival over Temodar alone. Although Accutane has shown to improve survival, it does have side effects, including dry skin and lips, headache, and nausea. It can also cause birth defects. An assay to detect the presence of EGFR on tumor cells is commercially available. Other drugs known to inhibit cell division through EGFR are also in development.

Thalidomide (Thalomid), another oral drug, is believed to inhibit growth of tumor cells by interfering with the tumor's ability to grow new blood vessels (anti-angiogenesis). Thalidomide was developed as a sedative in Europe, but was associated with devastating birth defects. It did not receive FDA approval until it was shown to be effective in treating leprosy. Thalidomide is effective in the treatment of a blood disorder, multiple myeloma, and has also been used in clinical trials for patients with malignant glioma. Used alone, it seems to slow the growth of tumors, although some patients experience tumor regression. Thalidomide has been used in combination with Temodar, CPT–11, and carboplatin. Its major side effects, sedation and constipation, are usually manageable. Both male and female patients are required to practice effective contraception while taking thalidomide.

Other commercially available drugs that may inhibit angiogenesis include the new cyclooxygenase–2 (COX-2) inhibitors, Vioxx and Celebrex, which are typically used to treat arthritis. In addition to treating arthritis, these drugs have shown to inhibit tumor growth in animal models. Both drugs have been used in the treatment of cancer, alone and in combination with chemotherapy. Side effects include nausea, headache, and stomach ulcers.

Tamoxifen (Nolvadex) has been used for several years in the treatment of breast cancer. When administered in higher doses, this drug has shown to be effective in the treatment of malignant glioma. It is believed that at higher doses tamoxifen inhibits a cell-signaling enzyme called protein kinase C, which prevents glioma cell division. Doses of tamoxifen used for treating brain tumor patients are 10 to 12 times higher than those commonly used for treating breast cancer.

Chemotherapy and Other Drug Therapy

Higher doses of tamoxifen may be associated with
deep vein thrombosis, the formation of blood clots in
the extremities (see Question 69). It may also cause
nausea, hot flashes, and weight gain. A recent study
suggested that patients on high-dose tamoxifen had an
improvement in survival when first treated with medication to reduce thyroid hormone production.

A number of other non-chemotherapy drugs are in
clinical trials. Because many are considerably less toxic
than chemotherapy, new combinations of non-
chemotherapy drugs and standard chemotherapy regimens appear promising.

52. How long should I stay on treatment?

The duration of treatment depends on many factors
but, ultimately, it depends on your response to treatment and the toxicity that you experience while on
treatment. Patients on clinical trials may have a specific duration of therapy planned as part of the trial or
may continue therapy as long as their tumor appears to
be responding. Some oncologists stop treatment after
the tumor has been in remission for at least two
months, but it is often difficult to determine whether
there is active tumor remaining.

Nitrosoureas such as BCNU and CCNU have
cumulative toxicity, sometimes causing prolonged
periods of low blood counts as treatment continues.
Both drugs may also be associated with lung scarring
(pulmonary fibrosis), which may be irreversible.
These drugs are rarely given for a year or more for
this reason. However, drugs such as Temodar, Procarbazine, and CPT–11 have been given for prolonged periods without significant cumulative

toxicity. Preliminary studies indicate that patients with malignant glioma who continue Temodar for longer than one year have an improvement in overall survival. Also, drugs such as Accutane, thalidomide, and tamoxifen may be taken without significant long-term toxicity, but no one knows the optimal duration of therapy.

53. Are all types of chemotherapy for brain tumors covered by insurance?

Private insurance, Medicare, and Medicaid may pay for some types of chemotherapy but not for others. For example, intravenous drugs such as BCNU may be covered by all three providers. Temodar is covered for primary brain tumors by most private insurers, and Medicare covers some—but not all—of the cost. However, off-label use of drugs may not be covered by Medicare or Medicaid. Even some private insurers may not cover a drug that is considered "experimental." Check with your doctor or your insurance company if you are unsure about whether your chemotherapy is covered.

54. Does oral chemotherapy have fewer side effects than intravenous chemotherapy?

The side effects of chemotherapy vary from person to person, and it is not always possible to predict their severity. Some oral drugs have similar side effects to intravenous drugs. For example, CCNU (oral) and BCNU (intravenous) both cause nausea and low blood cell counts. For patients who have had severe nausea and vomiting, BCNU may be a more appropriate choice because the drug is given in a vein. Patients who have vomiting after taking oral chemotherapy such as CCNU may thus receive less than the full dose intended.

Sometimes it may be difficult to find a suitable vein for the administration of chemotherapy. One problem that is avoided with oral chemotherapy is the insertion of an intravenous catheter.

Your oncologist will discuss with you the expected side effects of chemotherapy as well as how to manage the side effects if they occur.

55. Is it possible to get pregnant while on chemotherapy?

Yes—but it is very important to avoid pregnancy during chemotherapy and radiation therapy. Exposure to radiation therapy and chemotherapy, particularly early in pregnancy, is associated with a high risk to the fetus. Even later in pregnancy, chemotherapy may cause low birth weight and low blood counts in the unborn child.

Reliable contraception is recommended for all women of childbearing potential while undergoing treatment for a brain tumor. Chemotherapy can induce temporary or permanent infertility, and many female patients experience a change in their menstrual periods while receiving chemotherapy. Some patients experience premature menopause (their periods never return), and some resume their periods and normal fertility following chemotherapy.

A waiting period of several months following treatment with chemotherapy is also recommended for women who are considering pregnancy. This allows for recovery from the side effects of therapy. For women whose menstrual periods return to normal and are able to conceive, there does not appear to be an increased risk of birth defects.

56. If I return to work at my desk job while I'm on chemotherapy, will I have to take any special precautions?

Returning to work is a positive experience for many people who may have been away for several weeks after surgery or other treatment. However, most patients find that they are more fatigued than expected and may require more frequent breaks or a shorter work schedule. Even if you have a desk job, it is common to feel exhausted at the end of the day.

In addition to adequate rest, getting regular exercise and good nutrition are important for maintaining a sense of well-being while on chemotherapy. Patients who have nausea from their chemotherapy may be able to arrange their work schedules to allow more time off after chemotherapy. They may also be able to take nonsedating antiemetic medication.

Some patients on chemotherapy have low blood counts and are at risk for infection. Working closely with co-workers who may be ill or in rooms with poor ventilation may increase the risk of infection. Antibacterial soaps or hand wipes may help limit the transmission of infection in the workplace.

57. Will I lose my hair while on chemotherapy?

Although most people assume that hair loss is a universal side effect of chemotherapy, **alopecia** is actually uncommon with many of the drugs used to treat brain tumors. BCNU, CCNU, procarbazine, and Temodar usually do not cause hair loss. Drugs that may cause partial or complete hair loss include vincristine, CPT–11, Cytoxan, and etoposide.

Alopecia
hair loss.

PART SEVEN

Clinical Trials for Brain Tumor Patients

What is a clinical trial?

What do I need to know before I enroll in a study?

Are clinical trials only conducted at universities and research centers?

More . . .

58. My doctor told me that I'm "a perfect candidate for a clinical trial," but I'm not sure what he means by this. What is a clinical trial?

Clinical trial

a research protocol that is designed to answer a question regarding a population of patients with disease or who are at risk for disease.

A **clinical trial** is a study of patients with similar characteristics designed to answer a specific question or set of questions. Ideally, clinical trials study small populations, but they are intended to yield answers that may be applied to a larger population of similar patients. A clinical trial may study people who have not had a disease but are at risk for developing it. A clinical trial may test the effectiveness of a new drug or study a different way to give an older drug. A clinical trial may ask patients to give blood samples or tissue samples for testing after receiving different doses of a drug. A clinical trial may compare two different types of therapy in two sets of patients to determine which treatment is better tolerated or more effective. There are at least two components common to all clinical trials: (1) a written research plan, or **protocol,** written for the investigators conducting the study; and (2) the informed consent, which tells the patient what the clinical trial is designed to do and what he or she is expected to do as part of the study.

Protocol

a research plan for how a therapy is given is given and to whom it is given.

As in the examples above, not all clinical trials are designed to test new therapies. Although many new drugs or treatment strategies have been studied in a clinical trial, there are many questions unanswered because no clinical trial has yet studied them.

If your doctor has encouraged you to find out more about clinical trials, and said that you are a "perfect candidate," he is not only paying you a compliment, he's also telling you something about your medical condition. A patient who enters a clinical trial must be able to understand the principles of the trial he is considering. This does not mean that the patient needs a college degree, but it does mean that the patient should not have unrealistic expectations about the purpose of the trial and what the clinical trial will do for him as an individual. Clinical trials are not written for the benefit of individual patients; they are written to further the development of new treatments for a future population of patients. Also, patients who have severe medical problems that may interfere with the treatment on the trial are not eligible to participate in the study.

59. I'm interested in finding a clinical trial of a new treatment for glioblastoma multiforme. What do I need to know before I enroll in a study? Are clinical trials only conducted at universities and research centers?

Patients who are interested in enrolling in a clinical trial should be commended! Participation in a clinical trial can be time-consuming, inconvenient, and expensive, and patients are not paid for their participation. Some clinical trials may require frequent visits to a clinic or research center. Some trials may require more frequent testing than traditional therapy outside of a clinical trial. Some trials may require surgery or other invasive procedures. However, the only accurate way to answer questions about the side effects and effectiveness of new therapies is with a carefully conducted clinical trial.

There are several different types of clinical trials. A **pilot** or **feasibility study** is a small study of a new

Pilot study

small study designed to test an idea or treatment prior to a larger clinical trial; also called a feasibility study.

therapy or technology that may be very complicated or expensive. This type of study involves a small group of patients. It allows investigators to determine whether a larger trial should be performed. In some cases, the sponsor of a study (the organization that funds the research) will require that the new therapy show promise before allowing a large number of patients to receive it. An example of a pilot study is a trial that studies a group of brain tumor patients who are on the same therapy at two month intervals using MRI, PET, and a new imaging modality. The purpose of the study is to determine whether the new imaging technique provides additional information that may help predict the patient's response to therapy.

Preclinical studies are studies that use live animals to determine whether a particular treatment affects the heart, lungs, kidneys, and other organs. Animal models (animals with implanted tumors) are given the treatment to determine whether the treatment kills tumors without harming the animals. Other animal studies are conducted in normal animals to determine the effects of large doses of a drug. This type of study reveals the likely side effects that a human will experience after several months of taking the drug.

Preclinical study

study that uses live animals or cell cultures to determine the effectiveness and toxicity of a treatment.

Sample Preclinical Trial

Suppose that a new drug, YZ–1234, is discovered to kill human brain tumor cells in cell cultures. When administered to laboratory mice that have been implanted with human brain tumors, the tumors appear to shrink. YZ–1234 is then administered in larger doses to normal animals to determine its side effects. If any of the animals die after receiving the large doses of YZ–1234, their organs are studied to determine why they died. The results of these studies determine whether the drug is considered safe and effective enough to test in human subjects.

The Next Step

A **phase I trial** usually studies a small group of patients to determine whether a new treatment is safe for use in humans. Patients participating in a phase I study may not have the same type of tumor. In some cases, phase I studies are researching drugs that have not yet been studied in humans and the investigators begin the trial using a fraction of the dose found to be toxic in animals. As patients enter the trial, the doses of the drug are gradually escalated, with a careful review of side effects and laboratory tests. When side effects of the drug are noted more frequently or become more severe, the trial is stopped. Blood and urine tests are obtained during treatment to determine how the dose of the drug given correlates with the level of the drug in the blood and how rapidly the body excretes it. These studies, called **pharmacokinetics**, are very important in determining how toxic the drug may be in different patients and whether the drug can be used in patients who are taking other drugs. Remember that phase I trials rarely result in successful control of the patient's tumor. Even when the drug has been very effective in animal studies, the dose that can be tolerated in humans may not kill the tumor.

Phase I trial

study of a small group of patients to determine the side effects of a new treatment, with escalating intensity of the treatment administered.

Pharmacokinetics

study of how the body breaks down a drug after it is administered.

Sample Clinical Trial: Phase I

Back to our hypothetical new drug, which passed through preclinical studies: the next step is a phase I clinical trial. Patients entering this phase I clinical trial of the drug YZ–1234 receive one-tenth of the dose found to be toxic in mice. A small number of patients receiving YZ–1234 at the initial dose have no side effects, so the next group of patients receiving YZ–1234 receives a slightly higher dose. The trial continues until the patients receiving YZ–1234 show abnormalities in their blood tests or side effects that the investigators determine to be toxic but reversible. The YZ–1234 dose that the investigators find to be tolerable is 200 mg per day.

Phase II

Phase II trial

study of a group of similar patients to determine whether there is a statistical likelihood that a new treatment will be effective against a tumor.

A **phase II trial** studies a small group of patients, sometimes as few as 14, to determine whether there is a statistical likelihood that a new treatment will be effective against a specific tumor. If the study involves a drug, the dose that was determined to be safe for humans from the phase I trial will be used in all of the patients participating in the phase II trial. To determine whether the treatment is effective, it is important that all of the patients entered on a phase II trial are similar. Most phase II studies require that the patient have measurable disease because there must be a reference for determining whether the tumor is growing, shrinking, or remaining stable. The investigators may also choose to set **exclusion criteria,** which may limit the patient's number of previous treatments before entering the study. If the new treatment appears promising in a proportion of the initial patients, the study may be expanded to allow more patients to receive the drug.

Exclusion criteria

characteristics specified in a clinical trial that render the patient ineligible for the study.

A Sample Clinical Trial: Phase II

In a phase II trial of YZ–1234, the drug is given to 14 glioblastoma patients who have previously had surgery and radiation therapy and have evidence of tumor recurrence after radiation therapy. These patients receive 200 mg of YZ–1234 per day. After two months of treatment, three patients have evidence of tumor response (shrinkage), seven have no change, and four have evidence of tumor growth.

The Final Test: Phase III

A **phase III trial** compares two or more kinds of treatment in two or more similar groups of patients. Some phase III trials compare a new treatment that appeared promising in a phase II trial with the more standard therapy. Most phase III studies are **randomized trials,** meaning that the patients entering the trial are not given a choice of therapy. Instead, they are asked to accept a random chance of receiving either therapy. It is not known by either the investigators or the patients which arm of the trial contains the most effective therapy, although one arm may be less convenient, less toxic, or less expensive. Therefore, it is very important to determine whether there is a definite survival benefit in one arm over the other.

Some phase III trials are placebo-controlled, which would appear to be unfair to patients who are randomized to this group. A **placebo** often has the same appearance as the "real drug": the placebo may be a "sugar pill" of the same size and color or an intravenous solution of sugar water. However, some placebo-controlled trials offer the same effective therapy in both arms of the trial, with the new drug or placebo added to detect whether there is any additional benefit. This also allows investigators to determine whether there are subtle side effects of the new therapy. In a recent example, a placebo-controlled trial

Phase III trial

compares two or more kinds of treatment in two or more similar groups of patients, with one group of patients receiving the standard, or control, therapy.

Randomized trial

clinical trial involving at least two subgroups of patients comparing two or more different therapies, with the therapy selected by random assignment.

Placebo

a medication ("sugar pill") or treatment that has no effect on the body.

used the Gliadel wafer, which contains the chemotherapy drug carmustine, in one-half of the patients having surgery for glioblastoma. The other glioblastoma patients also had surgery and had a placebo wafer implanted that was identical in appearance to Gliadel. Neither the patients nor their surgeons knew which patients were receiving which wafers because all treatment was coded. At the end of the study, the investigators matched the patients with the treatment they received and determined that, on average, the patients who received Gliadel lived longer. This finding was very important to determine with a placebo-controlled study because all patients had some benefit just by removing the tumor.

Phase III studies are the largest, most time-consuming, and most expensive clinical trials to conduct. They often require hundreds of patients to detect statistical benefit. Many phase III studies involve multiple research centers and take several years to complete. Phase III studies may have an interim analysis stage, which is designed to detect differences in the two groups before the study has been completed. An interim analysis may suggest such a striking difference in the expected outcome of the patients in the two arms that the investigators decide to stop the study to avoid continuing to treat patients in the least effective way.

A Sample Clinical Trial: Phase III

The new drug YZ–1234 appears to be less toxic and at least as effective as some of the older treatments that have been used in glioblastoma. Therefore, a phase III study of 500 glioblastoma patients is planned. In this study, 250 of the patients will be randomized to receive radiation therapy followed by YZ–1234. The other

250 patients will receive radiation therapy followed by Temodar, which was chosen because it is also an oral drug. It is estimated that the study will take 2 to 3 years to complete.

Deciding to Join a Trial

Patients who are considering enrollment in a clinical trial should understand that clinical trials involve an element of risk. These risks are explained in the informed consent document. The patient should never sign an informed consent if he or she does not understand the question being posed in the clinical trial.

Often the study title contains the phase of the trial and the names of any drugs or treatments being used. For example, the title for the sample clinical trial discussed above would be: "A Phase I Study of YZ–1234 in Patients with Advanced Cancer." The known side effects of the therapy proposed in the clinical trial must be carefully stated in the informed consent. The informed consent usually states that unusual or unforeseen side effects may also occur. The treatment alternatives, including the standard treatments for the disease, must be stated. The investigators must also disclose whether enrollment in the clinical trial would affect the patient's enrollment in future clinical trials. Most clinical trials state that effective contraception must be practiced during treatment in a clinical trial because of a possible risk to an unborn child.

Enrollment in a clinical trial may be restricted to patients who are "minimally pretreated" because certain drugs may be more toxic to patients who have already had different types of chemotherapy. For this reason, if you are considering participation in a clinical trial, it is important to consider this early in treatment.

Many universities, regional cancer centers, and community cancer programs participate in clinical trials. Pharmaceutical companies sponsor some clinical trials, private foundations sponsor others, and still others are sponsored by the National Cancer Institute (NCI). The NCI provides financial support to cancer centers around the United States that participate in clinical research organizations, such as New Approaches to Brain Tumor Therapy (NABTT), Southwest Oncology Group (SWOG), and Eastern Cooperative Oncology Group (ECOG). In addition, the NCI conducts clinical trials at the National Institutes of Health Clinical Center in Bethesda, Maryland. Clinical trials that are supported by the NCI can be located on the Web at *www.cancer.gov/clinical_trials*. In addition, many individual cancer centers have Web sites that list their current clinical trials (see Question 100). Finally, Dr. Al Musella's web portal *www.virtualtrials.com* contains a very comprehensive listing of clinical trials for brain tumor patients.

60. What is the difference between an investigational therapy, an "off-label" drug, a complementary therapy, and an alternative therapy?

Investigational therapy

treatments that are experimental or under development in clinical trials, including drugs that were approved for other uses.

Investigational therapies or investigational drugs are treatments that are considered experimental or under development in a clinical trial setting. Some investigational drugs have not yet been approved for the treatment of any disease and cannot be obtained outside a clinical trial. Drugs that have been approved by the

Food and Drug Administration (FDA) for the treatment of one type of cancer may be considered investigational for the treatment of another type of cancer. Also, drugs that may be approved for intravenous use may be considered investigational when used by another route such as intra-arterially (injected directly into the artery supplying the tumor) or intrathecally (injected into the spinal fluid). Patients receiving investigational drugs on a clinical trial are allowed to continue taking the drug only if the treatment appears to be effective, as assessed by physical examination and scans. An investigational drug may be supplied free of charge to a patient who is enrolled in a clinical trial, but it is not always free, and the informed consent will specify this.

An off-label drug is approved by the FDA for one type of treatment but may be prescribed for other conditions. Some drugs may be both investigational and off-label. Because of the time required and the expense of performing clinical trials, only a small fraction of research studies are performed solely to obtain FDA approval for a drug. Some drugs that are widely accepted in brain tumor therapy, such as procarbazine and vincristine, have not been FDA-approved for this use. However, when clinical trials are published demonstrating that a treatment is effective and well-tolerated, doctors are more likely to prescribe the drug off-label. In some cases, insurance coverage does not reimburse for off-label use of the drug even when the patient's doctor determines that the drug is likely to be beneficial. You should always check with your doctor if you are concerned about whether the drug will be covered by your insurance.

Complementary treatment

treatment used in conjunction with standard treatment for disease.

Alternative therapy

treatment used in lieu of standard medical therapies.

Complementary therapies and **alternative therapies** encompass a wide variety of treatments, including herbal preparations, vitamin- or nutritional-based regimens, and therapeutic touch. Complementary therapies are used *in conjunction with* conventional therapy such as surgery, radiation therapy, and chemotherapy. Alternative therapies are used *in place of* conventional therapy. Some alternative therapies are based on the traditional medicines of other cultures, and others were developed by individual practitioners. A few alternative therapies have been studied in clinical trials. If you are interested in an alternative therapy, ask your doctor whether the treatment has been studied. It is also important to ask how long the treatment is expected to last because some alternative regimens cost hundreds or thousands of dollars a month. It has been estimated that up to 75% of all cancer patients use complementary or alternative therapy at some point during their illness.

Although investigational therapy and alternative therapy are both options for the patient who does not want conventional therapy, there are many differences between the two approaches. Doctors who offer the patient investigational therapy judge the patient's response to treatment by conventional means such as neurological examination and MRI. Patients enrolled in a clinical trial for an investigational therapy may be asked to forego all other treatments (including alternative therapies) that may interfere with the therapy being studied.

Alternative therapies may be prescribed by naturopaths or herbalists who are not licensed to practice medicine, and therefore they cannot order radiographic studies to determine response to treatment.

Some naturopathic practitioners follow the principle of complementary therapy. They allow chemotherapy or radiation treatment at the same time as the alternative therapy. Many insurance plans do not cover the costs of alternative therapy, even when it has been prescribed by a licensed physician.

61. I am interested in a clinical trial at a research center in another state, but my doctor is opposed to this. He wants me to enter a trial at the medical school in my city or take standard chemotherapy. What should I do?

There are many reasons why doctors do not refer their patients to clinical trials. If you have a good relationship with your local doctor and that doctor does not want you to participate in a particular clinical trial, make sure you ask why. If you are not happy with your doctor's answer, it is certainly possible to change doctors to find one who is more accepting of the clinical trial you want. Although it is possible to enter a clinical trial in another state without a referral from your doctor, you still need to have a local doctor in case of an emergency.

Some doctors feel that their patients assume that a clinical trial is better than standard therapy, but they know that the trial may not be successful. By definition, a new drug is being studied in a clinical trial because it has *not* proven superior to standard therapy. Moreover, less is known about a new drug than one that has already been studied and FDA approved. This is especially true when the clinical trial is a phase I study.

Some research centers have well-known doctors on staff or new treatments that have received national media attention. However, in most clinical trials only a few patients have the degree of success that is featured in the media. Your local doctor may be concerned that you are choosing a research center based on its reputation rather than its ability to offer you an appropriate treatment.

Some research centers manage the patient's care by having close communication with the local physician, and some do not. If the investigators running a clinical trial do not provide information about the investigational drug's side effects to a patient's local doctor, the local doctor is left "out of the loop." This may cause problems if the patient develops life-threatening complications related to the investigational drug, but the local physician has not been given any information about the side effects expected. If the patient comes to his hometown emergency room, the local doctor, not the research center doctor, will be called to see the patient. It is hardly surprising that the local physician will be unlikely to refer patients to that center in the future!

Some doctors feel that nearby medical schools should be supported in their research programs, and they may be more familiar with the investigators and the clinical trials offered at the local medical school. Your local doctor may also feel that frequent travel out of state will be more physically taxing on you than you realize.

It is best to schedule an appointment with your doctor to discuss your concerns. If you are considering conventional therapy after completion of the clinical trial, it is important to keep in touch with your local physician.

62. I have received three separate chemotherapy drugs, and each seemed to work for several months. I now have an area of new tumor on my MRI scan. I'm interested in a clinical trial, but several of the clinical trials I have seen don't allow patients who have had previous chemotherapy to participate. Why is this?

Clinical trials enroll patients who are very similar—to level the playing field, so to speak. In a phase II clinical trial, in which the objective of the trial is to test the effectiveness of a new drug, patients who have had no chemotherapy at all often respond better than patients who have had multiple types of chemotherapy. Investigators have a better chance of evaluating the promise of a new drug if patients who are "heavily pretreated" are not enrolled.

Often an objective of the clinical trial is to determine the potential side effects of a new treatment. When selecting participants for this type of trial, a patient's **bone marrow reserve** is an important factor. Bone marrow reserve is the term oncologists use to describe the expected recovery of the bone marrow cells—the cells that develop into the white blood cells, red blood cells, and platelets. This reserve is depleted when patients have had multiple treatment cycles of some chemotherapy drugs (particularly BCNU and CCNU). A patient whose bone marrow has been

Bone marrow reserve

term used by oncologists to describe the expectation of recovery of bone marrow cells following treatment with chemotherapy or radiation therapy.

depleted by previous chemotherapy may require platelet transfusions or growth factors such as Neupogen after every subsequent chemotherapy cycle to help the blood counts return to a normal level. If that patient is included in a clinical trial designed to study the side effects of a new treatment, the new drug may decrease blood cell counts to very low levels. The patient may require dose reductions of the new drug to continue chemotherapy, which may then lessen the chances that the new drug will be effective.

Very healthy patients with good bone marrow reserve are the favored subjects for clinical trial investigators who are hoping that a highly successful drug can be rapidly approved for general use. Again, it is important to remember that clinical trials are not written to benefit individual patients. They are written to develop new therapeutic strategies.

63. I have heard about a new treatment that's only available at a clinic overseas. It sounds promising, but how can I find out whether it's safe?

There are clinical trials in other countries that follow many of the same rules used for human research in the United States. Laws for the protection of human subjects guarantee that patients will be informed of the potential risks and benefits of participating in a clinical trial. Before considering a clinical trial that takes place in another country, you need to determine whether the treatment offered is funded by a research organization because private insurance probably will not cover the cost.

Clinical trials offered at research institutions in Europe may have reported their results at the Congress of the European Association for Neuro-Oncology. These **abstracts** can be reviewed by your local oncologist. If you are interested in participating (and you can afford it), your oncologist may be able to contact the principal investigator of the study to determine your eligibility. In some cases, a drug approved for cancer treatment overseas may be legally brought into the United States for treatment of an individual patient.

There are some drugs and therapies available in other countries that are not yet approved in the United States, but you should be careful to distinguish between investigational therapy and "unproven" therapy. "Unproven" therapy in other countries may be offered through "research clinics" that are little more than expensive resorts.

64. I have heard a lot about herbal remedies, shark cartilage, and other non-toxic treatments, but I was told that these treatments haven't been studied in a clinical trial. Is this true? If it is true, why haven't these treatments been studied?

There has been an explosion of interest in so-called non-toxic therapies. Patients interested in such therapy can now investigate them and participate in clinical trials at a number of sites. The National Institutes of Health's National Center for Complementary and Alternative Medicine (NCCAM) reports that an estimated $27 billion is spent on alternative and complementary therapies, such as herbal supplements, vitamins, plant

Abstract
brief summary of a scientific paper.

Clinical Trials for Brain Tumor Patients

extracts, shark cartilage, and hundreds of others. Some, but not all, supplements have been studied. Reviews of the results of these trials are now available.

Dr. Stephen Tomasovic, professor of molecular and cellular oncology at the MD Anderson Cancer Center, has compiled a list of complementary and alternative therapies and reviews of the scientific data, including the results of animal studies and clinical trials. This information is available on the web at *www.mdanderson.org/departments/CIMER*. The list includes traditional Chinese medicine, herbal and plant therapies, biologic agents, special diets, and energy therapies. In addition, the site contains information regarding drug interactions, a glossary of terms, and a "Frequently Asked Questions" section.

In the past, researchers who were interested in studying herbal supplements or nontraditional therapy had difficulty attracting funding for animal studies and clinical trials. There are now a number of sources of funding for such trials, including research grants through the National Institutes of Health. Patients who are interested in clinical trials for complementary and alternative therapies must be willing to forego other treatments while on the clinical trial to avoid confusing the results of the study.

M.L.'s comment:

Early on, my husband read about clinical trials on the Internet. Further research has indicated to us that clinical trials are a very good thing. Participation in a clinical trial was never offered to me, but I understand that my tumor, anaplastic oligodendroglioma, isn't as common, and there were no clinical trials in my area for newly diagnosed tumors. Because the majority of my tumor had been resected through surgery, I wouldn't have been eligible for phase II clinical trials. These trials require visible tumor to be present on a patient's MRI. My tumor responded so well to radiation therapy and chemotherapy that I still don't have enough visible tumor to qualify for a clinical trial ... but this is fine by me!

PART EIGHT

Complications of Brain Tumors and Their Treatment

Can I expect to have brain damage as a result of surgery, radiation therapy, or other treatment?

How long do I need to take anticonvulsant medication?

More ...

65. Can I expect to have brain damage as a result of surgery, radiation therapy, or other treatment?

A neurological deficit (a change in the brain that results in abnormal or reduced function) does not necessarily follow surgery or other therapy. The size and the location of your tumor may actually be creating a neurological deficit. This may improve when the tumor is removed and the pressure on the nearby brain structures returns to normal.

Neurosurgeons carefully evaluate the tumor's position in relation to the other brain structures. The type of surgery recommended is based on whether a permanent neurological deficit can be prevented. It is possible, however, that the tumor will be more difficult to remove than anticipated, or that bleeding or other complications will occur following surgery. The neurosurgeon will explain all of these risks to you before surgery.

The temporary disability that may occur after surgery, which often improves with rehabilitation, must be distinguished from the late effects of radiation therapy and chemotherapy. Although loss of strength or coordination is upsetting to some patients, intellectual decline and loss of short-term memory can be even more devastating. These effects on cognitive function may occur in patients who have achieved remission. Therefore, studying these effects must separate patients who have cognitive loss because of tumor progression.

Most studies of cognitive decline following brain tumor treatment have occurred in children. These children were long-term survivors (five years or longer) and most had received surgery and radiation therapy. Children who were younger at the time of diagnosis, who had larger radiation fields, and who had increased intracranial pressure at the time of diagnosis were found to be at increased risk for IQ loss and poor performance in school.

In one study of adults who survived primary and metastatic brain tumors at least one year, 12% suffered dementia and another 6% suffered psychological problems related to radiation therapy. Another study of adults treated for malignant brain tumors revealed that younger patients were more likely to improve over time, and most patients were able to return to their previous employment.

Patients at high risk for cognitive decline include those who are very young or very old at the time of diagnosis and treatment, those who have tumors of the cerebral hemispheres, and those who have radiation doses that include large daily fractions.

Although chemotherapy can also cause cognitive decline, it is difficult to separate the effects of chemotherapy from those caused by radiation therapy in patients who have received both types of treatment. Long-term survivors of primary CNS lymphoma have a higher rate of cognitive decline with chemotherapy and whole brain radiation therapy. High-dose chemotherapy paired with blood-brain barrier disruption, however, has not resulted in substantial intellectual impairment. This treatment success has increased the number of long-term survivors of primary CNS lymphoma, so recent research has focused on maintaining intellectual function in patients. As a result, a number of treatment protocols for CNS lymphoma have eliminated whole brain radiation therapy.

In most studies, it appears that aggressive treatment with either chemotherapy and radiation therapy or high doses of radiation therapy may yield the largest number of long-term survivors. Unfortunately, these treatment approaches also increase the risk for intellectual decline.

M.L.'s comment:

My husband and my parents were concerned that I would come out of brain surgery a changed person. When a person goes into the operating room for other types of surgery, he or she comes out physically changed, meaning the person may not have a bladder anymore or may no longer have a breast. The person's emotional state may be temporarily unstable, but the mind remains the same. When a person undergoes surgery on the brain, there is a fear that the person who comes out of the surgery won't be the same person who went in. Your brain controls all of your functions, such as memory, speech, and motor skills. If a tumor is in a location near any of these functional areas, there is a very good chance that you may not have the same essence that you once had. The thought that "you don't come out the way you went in" is every patient and caregiver's concern.

66. I experience short periods in which I can't speak. This happens several times a day. I never black out, but my neurologist says that I could be having seizures. Is this common?

About one-third of all brain tumor patients have seizures. These seizures may occur as the first symptom or may occur months or years after diagnosis.

Some tumor types are more commonly associated with seizures, particularly oligodendrogliomas. Seizures can be classified as partial or generalized.

Partial seizures originate from a specific area in the brain, often the area around the tumor. A partial seizure may have motor symptoms such as hand movement or sensory symptoms such as numbness or tingling. A simple partial seizure does not impair consciousness; a complex partial seizure does impair consciousness and the patient does not remember it.

Partial seizure

seizure involving only one area or lobe of the brain.

Generalized seizures involve both cerebral hemispheres and impair consciousness. A **tonic-clonic seizure**, often called **grand mal seizure,** involves spasm of the body limbs and trunk muscles, and the patient may have difficulty breathing. The patient loses consciousness during the seizure and is confused after the seizure. Weakness, muscle pain, and headache commonly occur following a tonic-clonic seizure.

Generalized seizure

seizure involving both hemispheres of the brain. Tonic-clonic or grand mal seizures are generalized seizures that include body spasms and breathing difficulties.

Status epilepticus, the continuation of a seizure or series of seizures without regaining consciousness, is a life-threatening condition. Patients with status epilepticus should be treated in an intensive care unit with intravenous medication and supplemental oxygen.

Status epilepticus

repeated seizures, or a seizure prolonged for at least 30 minutes.

An **electroencephalogram (EEG)** may be helpful in determining whether the episodes you experience are seizures; however, a normal EEG does not completely eliminate the possibility of a seizure disorder. In some hospitals, 24-hour EEG monitoring is available to determine whether a patient has infrequent seizures that may not be detected with a standard EEG.

Electroencephalogram (EEG)

a recording of the electrical impulses of the brain using electrodes attached to the scalp.

67. I had seizures before my tumor was diagnosed, but I haven't had one since. How long do I need to take anticonvulsant medication?

Certain types of tumors are more commonly associated with seizures. These include lower-grade tumors such as oligodendroglioma, astrocytoma, ganglioglioma, and dysembryoplastic neuroepithelial tumors. Occasionally, gross total resection of the tumor is possible and only short-term therapy with anticonvulsants is required, as long as the patient has remained seizure-free after the operation. Some patients can have surgical removal of both tumor and an adjacent area that is determined during the operation to be the origin of the seizures. This may also allow eventual discontinuation of anticonvulsant therapy.

For patients with residual tumor on MRI, anticonvulsant therapy should be continued. Tumor progression, drug interactions, and electrolyte imbalances can trigger further seizures, even when anticonvulsant drugs are used. It is extremely important to comply with your doctor's recommendations regarding anticonvulsant medication and follow-up. Never taper or discontinue your anticonvulsant medication without checking with your doctor.

68. Since the completion of my chemotherapy, I have noticed that I'm more short of breath. Why is this? Will this improve?

The pulmonary toxicity of some chemotherapy drugs, especially the nitrosoureas BCNU and CCNU, may not be apparent until months or even years later. Some patients have low-grade fever, cough, and shortness of breath on exertion, but their chest x ray may appear normal. Your doctor may order pulmonary function tests. These tests measure lung volumes, force of inhalation and exhalation, and gas exchange capability. A reduction in the gas exchange capability of the lung can be measured with a small amount of carbon monoxide. This is a sensitive test that determines whether the lung has developed scarring or fibrosis, a condition that prevents inhaled oxygen from reaching the red blood cells. Patients who develop symptoms of pulmonary fibrosis can be treated with oral steroid therapy (prednisone) for several weeks. Some patients require supplemental oxygen. Although the risk of developing pulmonary toxicity from BCNU or CCNU is higher with multiple cycles of therapy, patients who had lung disease or who smoked before treatment with chemotherapy may develop toxicity earlier. Other drugs that may cause lung toxicity include bleomycin, methotrexate, cyclophosphamide, and procarbazine.

Pulmonary toxicity can be disabling or fatal, even in long-term survivors of brain tumors. Monitoring symptoms and pulmonary function tests may help detect early signs of pulmonary fibrosis so that treatment can be modified if needed. However, treatment modification may involve stopping the therapy that is effective in controlling the tumor.

69. Over the past several days, I have noticed that my left leg seems swollen and tight compared to my right. When I called my oncologist's office and talked to the nurse, she told me to go to the

emergency room immediately. What's the problem? Why do I have to go to the ER?

The nurse is concerned that you may have a deep vein thrombosis (DVT), a blood clot in a large vein. The large veins of the legs may develop long, thick clots that block the return of blood flow to the heart. This can cause pain and swelling. The most dangerous complication of a DVT, however, occurs if the clot breaks away from the walls of the vein and travels to the heart. A large clot can become lodged in the heart valves, but more commonly the clot becomes lodged in the arteries of the lung. A clot that has clogged the pulmonary arteries is called a **pulmonary embolus**. A pulmonary embolus can cause sudden death. It has been estimated that up to 15% of all cancer patients die of pulmonary embolus.

Although DVT does not always result in pulmonary embolus, the presence of a clot in the extremities should be taken very seriously. Doctors hospitalize patients with DVT to keep them at bed rest, to begin anticoagulant therapy, and to evaluate further for evidence of pulmonary embolus.

A DVT in the lower limbs can be detected by ultrasound, which can detect blood flow through the veins below the surface of the skin and muscle. The most dangerous clots are those in the deep veins of the thigh and pelvis because these vessels are quite large.

A pulmonary embolus does not always cause symptoms. Some clots break up gradually, releasing a shower of small clots that lodge in the pulmonary ves-

Pulmonary embolus

blood clot that travels through the veins and through the heart, eventually blocking one or more pulmonary arteries.

146

sels. A large clot typically causes shortness of breath, chest pain, or cough. Although a chest x ray may be normal, other tests, such as a ventilation/perfusion scan or a chest CT angiogram, may show a loss of normal blood flow to one or both lungs. Patients may require supplemental oxygen for several days because of this blockage of blood flow to the lung.

Anticoagulants (blood thinners), such as heparin, enoxaparin (Lovenox), dalteparin (Fragmin), and tinzaparin (Innohep), prevent the development of further clots. However, these drugs are all given by injection. Many patients prefer to take an oral anticoagulant called warfarin (Coumadin). Patients taking warfarin must be closely monitored with regular blood tests because of the drug's interactions with other medications and certain foods.

Some DVT patients, including those with recent neurosurgery, are at risk for bleeding complications from anticoagulants. Such patients may benefit from placement of an inferior vena cava (IVC) filter, which is an internal device that is placed into the large vein below the heart to act as a screen for blood clots that may break off and travel to the heart and lungs. An IVC filter is often used in combination with an anticoagulant because DVT may still form in the limbs, causing pain and swelling.

It is not always possible to predict or prevent DVT. Patients who are not ambulatory, who have had recent surgery, and who have a history of DVT should discuss ways to reduce the risk of DVT and pulmonary embolus with their doctors.

70. Are infections more common in patients with brain tumors?

Brain tumor patients are not necessarily more suscepti-
ble to infection as a result of the tumor; however, their
treatment may place them at risk for certain kinds of
infections. Many brain tumor patients are treated with
steroids such as dexamethasone before and after surgery. A short course of steroids usually does not increase
the risk of infection. However, long-term steroid use
(over a period of weeks or months) is often associated
with fungal infections, particularly oral thrush (candidiasis). Thrush appears as a white coating over the tongue
and back of the throat, and although it may be painless,
it can affect taste and appetite. Extensive candidiasis of
the esophagus and genitourinary tract may be painful
and require several days of oral antifungal therapy.

Some chemotherapy drugs, especially when used in
combination with steroids, increase the risk of infection. Temodar, a drug that usually is not associated
with a low white blood cell count, affects the subset of
white cells called lymphocytes that are important in
preventing fungal and viral infections. Serious lung
infections, including *Pneumocystis carinii*, *Aspergillus*,
and *Nocardia*, are rare in the normal population but are
life-threatening in patients with low lymphocyte
counts. Patients who have a history of herpes infections may also experience an increase in the number
and severity of outbreaks.

Patients who develop a low neutrophil count (see
Question 44) as a result of chemotherapy must take
precautions to avoid infection and notify their doctors
immediately for fever, chest congestion, or cough.

Patients who have implanted intravenous catheters for administering chemotherapy are at risk for infection and should notify their doctor if they experience any tenderness around the catheter, fever, or chills.

71. Will my cancer treatments cause permanent infertility?

A number of different chemotherapy drugs can cause premature menopause, irregular menstrual periods, and infertility in women. Chemotherapy drugs can also cause infertility in men. Procarbazine, Temodar, cisplatin, and carboplatin have been associated with sterility. For some patients, the sterility is only temporary, and they recover fertility within a year after stopping treatment. However, permanent sterility is more common in men, and in women who are older than age 40 at the time of treatment.

Brain radiation can decrease or destroy the normal production of hormones that affect sexual development and reproduction. Men may benefit from testosterone injections to improve libido, decrease hot flashes, and prevent osteoporosis. Similarly, women who experience premature menopause after radiation therapy may benefit from low-dose estrogen and progesterone replacement therapy. Such therapy is usually prescribed to alleviate symptoms rather than to restore fertility.

Male patients who desire to father children following treatment may be able to bank sperm before starting therapy. For female patients, preservation and harvesting of eggs requires considerably more time and expense. The need to initiate therapy as soon as possible may not provide enough time to retrieve viable eggs.

Some patients with pituitary tumors, or tumors in areas near the pituitary, may have abnormal sex hormone production at diagnosis. Disrupted hormone production may cause ovarian or testicular failure, resulting in infertility. These patients therefore cannot benefit from fertility preservation strategies before chemotherapy.

72. I've always been healthy, but now that I have a brain tumor I worry about every little symptom. What are the symptoms I should look for, and when should I call my doctor?

It's not always easy to know *when* to call your doctor, or even *which* doctor to call. Some problems can wait until your doctor can see you in the outpatient clinic, and some need immediate attention. At night or on the weekend, your doctor may direct you to the emergency room. Make sure you follow your doctor's recommendation.

If you've just had surgery, your neurosurgeon will want you to report any changes in your condition following your discharge from the hospital. If you experience infection in the surgical wound, fever higher than 100°F, sudden onset of headache, or increasing weakness, call your neurosurgeon.

If you are seeing a neurologist for seizures, this doctor will manage your anticonvulsant medication and monitor any laboratory tests that might be required. Don't expect your other doctors to adjust your anticonvulsant medications. Your neurologist is expected to take charge in this area and will make any medication adjustments.

Your radiation oncologist will typically see you at least once a week during your treatment. After therapy is completed, most radiation oncologists release you back to the care of your neurosurgeon, oncologist, or neurologist. If you develop a complication that requires admission to a hospital while you are receiving radiation therapy, let your radiation oncologist know. It may be possible to continue your treatment while hospitalized.

In many communities, a medical oncologist or neuro-oncologist assumes the care of a brain tumor patient after surgery. The medical oncologist or neuro-oncologist will work with the other specialists and your primary care doctor to arrange any laboratory tests or radiographic studies that you need. Although your primary care doctor may still treat other medical problems unrelated to the tumor (such as high blood pressure and diabetes), your oncologist will address the treatment of the brain tumor and any complications related to the tumor. Table 5 provides a list of what you need to bring to your oncologist's attention immediately.

On the other hand, there are situations for which you *should not* call your oncologist in the middle of the night. For example, a refill on your cholesterol medication, the results of an MRI scan taken earlier in the day, or a question about chemotherapy you received last month are *not* considered emergencies. Keep in mind that your doctor (or the partner who may be on

Table 5   Problems to report to your oncologist

Problem	Possible Causes/Concerns
Sudden shortness of breath or chest pain	Pulmonary embolus or heart attack
Fever of 100°F or higher, especially when accompanied by chills	Severe infection
Swelling in one or both legs	Deep vein thrombosis
Severe nausea and vomiting or diarrhea	Could result in dehydration
Sudden onset of severe headache	Brain hemorrhage
Vomiting brown fluid or blood	Bleeding ulcer
Seizures that rapidly recur over a period of minutes	Onset of status epilepticus
Severe rash, especially one that involves the mouth or rectum	Life-threatening drug reaction
Numerous tiny red spots over the legs, bleeding gums	Low platelet count

call) will not have access to your medical record after office hours.

Make sure you keep a card with all of your doctors' names and phone numbers available in your wallet or purse in the event that another doctor needs to contact one of them regarding your care.

PART NINE

Medications Used in Brain Tumor Treatment

What does dexamethasone do? What are the side effects of dexamethasone?

What are the side effects of anticonvulsant medication?

More ...

73. After surgery, I was prescribed dexamethasone. My doctor says I may be on this drug several days. What does dexamethasone do? What are the side effects of dexamethasone?

Corticosteroid

a naturally occurring hormone produced by the adrenal cortex, or a synthetic hormone having similar properties; often used to treat edema (swelling) in leaky capillaries of the brain.

Dexamethasone (Decadron) is a **corticosteroid,** a medication that reduces edema (swelling) around brain tumors by decreasing the tendency of fluid to leak from the blood vessels into the surrounding brain tissue. In addition to its effects in reducing edema, it is often used with chemotherapy to control nausea and vomiting. Dexamethasone is available as an intravenous form or in tablets.

Most brain tumor patients are given dexamethasone before surgery, and many have noticed improvement in their symptoms within days of beginning treatment with dexamethasone. However, high doses of dexamethasone cannot be continued indefinitely because of the side effects that tend to become more pronounced with a longer duration of therapy.

Because dexamethasone suppresses normal hormone production by the adrenal gland, serious side effects can occur if you suddenly stop taking it. Follow your doctor's instructions exactly when taking dexamethasone or when tapering off of it.

The side effects of dexamethasone vary with the dose and duration of use, and also from patient to patient. Some of the most common side effects include weight gain, heartburn, fluid retention, muscle weakness, increased appetite, osteoporosis, insomnia, depression, nervousness, mania/mood swings, high blood sugar, low potassium, high blood pressure, thinning hair, rash or acne, thin skin, increased risk of infection, and cataracts.

Rapid withdrawal of dexamethasone may cause muscle and joint aches, low blood pressure, loss of appetite, nausea and vomiting, low-grade fever, and headache. Sometimes it is necessary to continue the dose of dexamethasone at a constant level for a longer period of time to allow recovery from steroid withdrawal symptoms. After recovery, your doctor will try to taper the drug at a slower rate.

Dexamethasone also can interact with many drugs, including anticonvulsants such as phenytoin (Dilantin) and phenobarbitol. Dexamethasone may cause stomach upset when given with aspirin or nonsteroidal anti-inflammatory drugs such as ibuprofen (Advil).

M.L.'s comment:

When I was taking Decadron, the primary side effect that I experienced was weight gain. Just about everyone I know that has taken Decadron (or any steroid) has also experienced weight gain. Most people don't like to gain weight (myself included). To go through this experience is very frustrating; however, I had to just "suck it up" and realize that this was part of being sick. Frankly, I was happy to be alive, but the weight gain still bothered me at times. I think it's OK to be frustrated when the weight gain occurs, just as long as you don't let the frustration consume you. I have seen other patients' attitudes become so negative because of their weight gain. This isn't healthy. Just remember, the weight WILL COME OFF! I promise! I gained about 20 pounds or more and eventually it all came off. I really had to work at losing the last 5 pounds, but I did lose it.

74. What are the side effects of anticonvulsant medication?

There are common, expected side effects of anticonvulsant medication, and rare, life-threatening side effects. Follow your doctor's instructions exactly when taking anticonvulsants. Many of these drugs must be closely monitored with blood tests. Table 6 is a list of common anticonvulsant drugs, their common side effects, and the rare but serious side effects that sometimes occur.

M.L.'s comment:

The side effects of anticonvulsant medication can vary depending on the kind that you're taking. For example, I took Dilantin for about 15 months and the primary side effect that I experienced was fatigue. It's my understanding that this is a fairly common side effect to expect, and the extent of the fatigue will vary by individual. My neurologist was able to prescribe another medication called Provigil to assist with the fatigue that I experienced while on Dilantin. My husband called it my "picker upper" because that is exactly what it did. It really was wonderful in giving my body that boost of energy and it kept me from feeling so tired at the end of the day.

I recently changed from Dilantin to a different medication called Keppra. Keppra is really wonderful because it doesn't cause the same level of fatigue that I was feeling with the Dilantin. In fact, I have been able to stop using the Provigil that I was taking on a daily basis with the Dilantin.

My recommendation is that you talk to your neurologist regularly about how your anticonvulsant medications are making you feel because the side effects can vary with each

Table 6 Side effects of anticonvulsant medication

Common Name	Generic Name	Common Side Effects	Rare Side Effects
Depakote	Valproic acid	Drowsiness, nausea, tremor, weight gain	Pancreatitis, hepatitis
Dilantin	Phenytoin	Drowsiness, skin rash, dizziness, thickening of gums	Hepatitis, low blood counts, enlarged lymph nodes, severe skin reaction
Gabitril	Tiagabine	Drowsiness, dizziness, fatigue, nervousness	Lethargy, poor responsiveness
Keppra	Levetiracetam	Drowsiness, fatigue, dizziness	
Lamictal	Lamotrigine	Drowsiness, skin rash, fatigue	In children, more severe skin rash which may be life-threatening
Neurontin	Gabapentin	Drowsiness, dizziness, fatigue	Visual disturbances, nausea, rash, tremor
Phenobarbitol	Phenobarbitol	Drowsiness, impaired cognition, reduced libido, depression	Hyperactivity, behavior changes
Tegretol	Carbamazepine	Drowsiness, dizziness, double vision, low blood counts, skin rash	Visual disturbances, depression, loss of coordination
Topamax	Topiramate	Drowsiness, fatigue, psychomotor slowing, weight loss	Speech disorders, kidney stones
Trileptal	Oxcarbazepine	Drowsiness, dizziness, rash	Double vision, loss of coordination
Zonegran	Zonisamide	Drowsiness, dizziness, loss of appetite, nausea, weight loss	Kidney stones

person. There are other medications that can be prescribed in an effort to assist with your particular needs.

Here's a few tips that help me boost my energy when I'm feeling tired:

- When possible try to incorporate some activity into your schedule. Even a short walk around the block will help get your blood moving and will give your body more energy.
- Take frequent breaks whenever possible.
- Eat as nutritiously as possible, and don't be afraid to eat. Food gives your body the fuel it needs to keep going.
- If a task doesn't have to be done right away, either don't do it or have someone else do it for you.
- Give yourself permission to stop when you're feeling tired. Take a nap if you need one. Listen to your body and realize that it's OK to allow yourself to take it slow.

75. My pharmacist said that there may be a "drug interaction" between some of my medications. What does this mean?

Many drugs undergo chemical changes in the body after intravenous or oral administration. When different drugs are used at the same time, one drug may affect the normal action of the other. Some drugs are chemically processed in the liver, but another drug used simultaneously may affect the normal processing of the first drug. In the case of both chemotherapy drugs and anticonvulsant drugs, the amount of the drug needed to produce the desired effect without toxicity (the therapeutic level) is very important.

Anticonvulsant drug interactions are particularly critical because the patient may have seizures if the therapeutic level drops. Some drugs will raise the anticonvulsant drug level, possibly resulting in a toxic level. Also, the use of an anticonvulsant drug may render the other drug partially or completely ineffective. Your pharmacist is trained to examine the list of your medications and look for possible drug interactions with your anticonvulsant.

A brief list of common drug interactions with anticonvulsants is given in Table 7.

Chemotherapy can also interact with other medications. Table 8 lists the most common interactions of chemotherapy drugs.

76. My primary care doctor prescribed a medication for my sinus infection. Do I have to tell my oncologist about this drug because I'm on chemotherapy?

Yes. It's a good idea to make sure your doctors know about any changes in your medication, not only because of the possibility of drug interactions, but because of the reason a new drug was prescribed in the first place. Your oncologist will want to know if you have *any* signs or symptoms of infection while you are taking chemotherapy. He may delay your next chemotherapy course until you recover from an infection. Your oncologist will also want to closely follow

Table 7 Drug interactions with anticonvulsant medications

Anticonvulsant	Will Raise Anticonvulsant Level	Will Lower Anticonvulsant Level	Other Drug Effects
Dilantin	Topamax, Tagamet, Bactrim, Diflucan, Zantac, Prozac, Prilosec, Coumadin	Tegretol, Phenobarbitol, Depakote, some chemotherapy drugs	Decreases effectiveness of oral contraceptives (OCPs), Coumadin, some antibiotics, antifungals and HIV drugs, steroids
Tegretol	Erythromycin, Darvocet, Tagamet, Cardizem, Prozac, Zoloft, Verapamil	Phenobarbitol, Dilantin	Decreases effectiveness of OCPs, antifungals, Demerol
Depakote		Tegretol, Phenobarbital, Dilantin, Aspirin	Increases sedation when used with Xanax, Vicodin, Demerol, Fioricet, Darvocet, Phenergan
Phenobarbital		Dilantin, Tegretol	Similar to Dilantin
Zonegran	Lamictal	Tegretol, Dilantin, Phenobarbital	

(continued)

Medications Used in Brain Tumor Treatment

Table 7   Drug Interactions with anticonvulsant medications (continued)

Anticonvulsant	Will Raise Anticonvulsant Level	Will Lower Anticonvulsant Level	Other Drug Effects
Trileptal		Dilantin, Tegretol, Phenobarbital	Decreases effectiveness of OCPs; similar to Tegretol
Lamictal	Depakote	Dilantin, Tegretol	May interact with methotrexate, Bactrim
Topamax		Dilantin, Tegretol	Decreases effectiveness of OCPs; increased sedative effect with narcotics, tranquilizers
Gabatril		Dilantin, Tegretol, Phenobarbitol	Increased sedative effect with narcotics, tranquilizers, Phenergan

Table 8 Interactions of Chemotherapy with Other Treatments

Chemotherapy Drug	Interacts With	Result of Interaction
BCNU (Carmustine) and CCNU (Lomustine)	Radiation Therapy	Lower blood counts than BCNU alone
	Bone marrow depressants (chemotherapy, AZT, Amphotericin B)	Lower blood counts than BCNU alone
	Live virus vaccine	Increased side effects of vaccine; may have poor response to vaccination
Procarbazine (Matulane)	Killed virus vaccine	Poor response to vaccination
	Alcohol	CNS depression; possible hypertensive reaction
	Cocaine	Severe hypertension
	Anesthesia, spinal	Severe hypotension
	Antihistamines	Gastrointestinal effects
	Anticonvulsants	Increased CNS depression
	Oral hypoglycemics	Enhances hypoglycemic effects
	Caffeine	Cardiac arrhythmias, hypertension
	Antidepressants (Prozac, Elavil, Buspar)	Confusion, agitation, severe hypertension, seizures
	Demerol, other narcotics	Excitation, rigidity, hypertension
	Live virus vaccine	See BCNU, above
	Killed virus vaccine	See BCNU, above

(continued)

162

Table 8   Interactions of Chemotherapy with Other Treatments (continued)

Chemotherapy Drug	Interacts With	Result of Interaction
Temodar (Temozolomide)	Depakote	No definite clinical effects; possibly prolongs toxicity of Temodar
	BCNU, CCNU	Lowers blood counts more than would be expected for either drug alone
	Live virus vaccine	See BCNU, above
	Killed virus vaccine	See BCNU, above
Etoposide (VP–16)	Cyclosporin	Increases toxicity of etoposide
	Radiation Therapy	Lowers blood counts more than expected for etoposide alone
	Live virus vaccine	See BCNU, above
	Killed virus vaccine	See BCNU, above
CPT–11 (Camptosar, irinotecan)	Radiation Therapy	Lowers blood counts more than expected for CPT–11 alone
	Dexamethasone	May result in lower lymphocyte counts
	Diuretics (Lasix, Dyazide)	May increase risk of dehydration
	Oral Hypoglycemic Agents	May increase hyperglycemia, particularly when CPT–11 is given with dexamethasone
	Chemotherapy (many)	May increase toxicity of CPT–11
	Laxatives	Decreases blood levels of CPT–11, reducing effectiveness
	Dilantin	May worsen CPT–11–related diarrhea
	Live virus vaccine	See BCNU, above
	Killed virus vaccine	See BCNU, above

(continued)

Table 8 Interactions of Chemotherapy with Other Treatments (continued)

Chemotherapy Drug	Interacts With	Result of Interaction
Carboplatin (Paraplatin)	Radiation Therapy	Lowers blood counts more than expected for carboplatin alone
	Cisplatin	Previous treatment with cisplatin may increase risk of neurotoxicity and hearing loss
	Aminoglycoside antibiotics (Gentamicin, Amikacin, Tobramycin)	May increase risk of renal toxicity and hearing loss
	Live virus vaccine	See BCNU, above
	Killed virus vaccine	See BCNU, above
Cisplatin (Platinol)	Radiation Therapy	May increase toxicity; dose reduction recommended
	Aminoglycoside antibiotics	See carboplatin, above
	Tegretol	May reduce blood levels
	Depakote	May reduce blood levels
	Dilantin	May reduce blood levels
	Topamax	May reduce blood levels
	Phenobarbitol	May reduce blood levels
	Lamictal	May reduce blood levels
	Gabatril	May reduce blood levels
	Antivert, Compazine, Thorazine, Antihistamines	Concurrent use may mask cisplatin-induced toxicity
	Bleomycin	Cisplatin-induced renal impairment may increase toxicity of bleomycin
	Live virus vaccine	See BCNU, above
	Killed virus vaccine	See BCNU, above

(continued)

Medications Used in Brain Tumor Treatment

Table 8   Interactions of Chemotherapy with Other Treatments (continued)

Chemotherapy Drug	Interacts With	Result of Interaction
Methotrexate	Alcohol	May increase liver toxicity
	Coumadin	Increases effect; may increase risk of hemorrhage
	Non-steroidal anti-inflammatory drugs (NSAIDs); Aspirin	May increase methotrexate toxicity
	Radiation Therapy	Lower blood counts; may cause increased neurotoxicity during whole brain radiation
	Dilantin	Increases methotrexate toxicity
	Penicillins	Increases methotrexate toxicity
	Accutane	Increases liver toxicity
	Oral hypoglycemic agents	Increases methotrexate toxicity
	Bactrim, Trimethoprim-Sulfamethoxazole	Lower blood counts with concurrent treatment
	Live virus vaccine	See BCNU, above
	Killed virus vaccine	See BCNU, above
Vincristine (Oncovin)	Dilantin	Reduces blood levels, with possible increase in seizure risk
	Sporonox	Increased severity of neuromuscular side effects
	Spinal cord irradiation	May produce additive neurotoxicity
	Live virus vaccine	See BCNU, above
	Killed virus vaccine	See BCNU, above

your white blood cell count because an infection can be more serious if the white blood cell count is low.

77. I've never been depressed before, but since my diagnosis I feel hopeless at times. Will an antidepressant help? Are there side effects that I need to consider if I'm on chemotherapy?

Depression in brain tumor patients can be related to the stress of the diagnosis and treatment, the loss of physical or mental capabilities, and the fear of suffering and death. For patients who have always enjoyed good health, the diagnosis of a brain tumor can be emotionally overwhelming. Almost all patients who are faced with serious illness experience at least temporary grief and anxiety about their condition, but there are some patients who become so distraught that they are unable to make decisions regarding their own care. These patients may benefit from counseling or supportive psychotherapy with a medical professional experienced in helping patients with severe illness.

Severely depressed patients and patients with milder forms of depression may benefit from antidepressant medication. Some of the newer antidepressant drugs, known as selective serotonin reuptake inhibitors (SSRIs), include fluoxetine (Prozac), sertraline (Zoloft), paroxetine (Paxil), and citalopram (Celexa). These drugs have fewer side effects than the older tricyclic antidepressants such as amitriptyline (Elavil) and nortriptyline (Pamelor). Moreover, tricyclic antidepressants may increase the risk of seizures in some patients. Another antidepressant, bupropion (Wellbutrin; also known as Zyban when prescribed for smoking cessation) also increases the risk of seizures.

Patients who are taking procarbazine chemotherapy (one of the components of the popular combination PCV) need to be aware of potential drug interactions with antidepressant medications. Neither the SSRI drugs nor tricyclic antidepressants should be used by patients taking procarbazine.

Some patients resist the idea of taking antidepressant medication because of the large number of other medications they must take. However, studies have shown that cancer patients have an improvement in their overall quality of life when treated for depression. Studies also show that patients treated with antidepressants experience an increase in the number of natural killer cells, the cells that have an important role in the immune system.

78. Can I drink alcohol while taking chemotherapy or anti-seizure medication?

There are some drugs used in brain tumor therapy that have known toxic reactions with alcohol; these include procarbazine, methotrexate, and thalidomide. Alcohol can interact with many other medications, including anticonvulsants, antidepressants, tranquilizers, sleeping pills, and pain medications. These drugs enhance the effect of alcohol, and therefore driving, even after very small amounts of alcohol, should be strictly forbidden. Patients taking anticonvulsants who also drink may experience wide fluctuations in drug levels, creating a risk of seizures or toxicity.

Many patients can drink a glass of champagne at a wedding or sip a pina colada on the beach without risk, but regular use of alcohol should be avoided when taking the medications listed above.

M.L.'s comment:

Personally, I would recommend that you NOT drink alcohol while taking chemotherapy. First of all, depending on the type of chemotherapy that you're taking, you'll probably experience fatigue as a side effect. Coupling alcohol with chemotherapy will make you even more tired. If you're like most people, you may experience fatigue with your anti-seizure medication, and mixing alcohol with it will make you feel that much worse.

PART TEN

Living With a Brain Tumor

I have just learned that I have a brain tumor and I'm afraid. Is this common?

Are feelings of anger and depression normal reactions to the diagnosis of a brain tumor?

What dietary adjustments do I need to make during treatment?

More ...

79. I have just learned that I have a brain tumor and I'm afraid. Is this common?

Yes. Most people who are diagnosed with serious illness grapple with fear and anxiety. Some patients fear physical disability, loss of income, loss of health insurance, or loss of support from their family. Some patients fear surgery, radiation therapy, or other treatment. Some patients fear that they will die. The majority of people fear what they cannot control, and there are many aspects of brain tumors that are unpredictable and uncontrollable.

Not all brain tumors are life-threatening. Some can be cured surgically, and some can be controlled for long periods of time with radiation therapy or chemotherapy. Learning about your condition may help you cope with your fear. If you fear specific aspects of your treatment, tell your doctor so that you can receive help in coping with your treatment.

M.L.'s comment:

If you aren't afraid, then you aren't normal! I was feeling great; I was about to get promoted to vice-president. My husband and I were talking about starting a family. I didn't have any warning signs at all. Then I woke up one morning and I didn't feel well. The next thing I knew, I was told that I had a brain tumor. Frankly, I didn't know what that really meant. My husband did a great deal of research on the Internet to find out as much as he could about brain tumors. I was scared, but there seemed to be this voice inside of me that kept telling me that I would be OK. I had read at one time that "cancer is NOT a death sentence" and I believed that.

Having faith in God and believing I would be taken care of also helped ease my fears. Someone told me once that faith was the most effective antidote for fear. That proved to be true in my situation. Others have suggested that hope is the most effective antidote for fear. I'm sure there are many different opinions about what is considered effective for fighting the battle with cancer. I just continued to believe that I would be OK and that I would make it through all of this.

My husband, friends, and family were all an incredible support system for me. Believe me, I was depressed at times, too. There were times when I cried a lot. About 3 or 4 months after my surgery—when I was well into my radiation treatments—I seemed to be very emotional for a period of several weeks. When my mother or my sister, Annemarie, would call me to see how I was doing, I would just start to cry. I think the reality of the situation had set in. My doctors told me that the depression could have also been associated with my medication.

80. Are feelings of anger and depression normal reactions to the diagnosis of a brain tumor? What other feelings should I expect to experience?

M.L.'s comment:

Based on everything that I have either felt myself, read elsewhere, or heard from others, it's perfectly natural to have negative feelings about the diagnosis that you've been given. You have to deal with the fact that your life has changed. You'll probably experience other feelings, such as denial and resentment. During the initial stages, you'll probably become somewhat numb to it all. Again, all of this is normal. I experienced all of these feelings; however, at some point after the reality of the situation set in, I realized how important it was for me to think about how I could take those negative feelings and turn them into positive energy. For some reason, I kept thinking that this happened to me for a reason. My husband kept thinking, "Why M.L.?" and "What has she done in her life to deserve this?" Eventually, a sense of acceptance set in that changed the way we lived our lives from that moment on. Duane and I did talk openly about my diagnosis and how it changed our lives. I needed him to tell me many of the details that took place early on because I couldn't remember them. Duane was (and still is) terrified that he was going to lose me within the first year of my diagnosis. I felt like I had to be strong for him because he was so worried that he would lose me. I think the thought of me not being the "same M.L." scared him almost as much as the thought of losing me completely. We talked about all of these feelings, and we allowed ourselves to be unhappy while we were having these discussions. We always tried to end such discussions on a positive note. We'd say that we would fight this one day at a time and deal with whatever was given to us.

This whole situation actually brought Duane and I closer. We were very close before, but coping with news of this magnitude was something that neither of us had ever had to do. We found that we clung to one another for support and strength. I also found a great deal of comfort and strength in my religion. The church and my pastor, Father Henry, were there for me and prayed for me all the time. I can't even begin to tell you how many people told me they were praying for me, and I believe that a person who gets prayed for gets well more quickly.

Since my diagnosis, I feel like my personal life has changed for the better. I've heard others say the same thing. I think

*it's because you're forced to take a good look at how your life
was before the diagnosis of a brain tumor. You're given a
chance to re-evaluate your life and make changes for the
better. I started trying to figure out what "message was
being sent to me" and what I was supposed to do with the
message I received. I sometimes wonder if this all happened
because it was a way to get me to help other people with
brain tumors. By sharing my story of dealing with a
malignant brain tumor, I could help others be more positive
about their situations. I've thought about this so many
times, and every time I get a different answer. These days,
I just try to do the best I can to live a good life. I try to be a
good influence on others who may be coping with some of
the same issues that I experienced with a brain tumor.*

81. What dietary adjustments do I need to make during treatment? Should I take vitamin or mineral supplements? Can diet protect against recurrence of a brain tumor?

Dietary adjustments may be necessary, but recommendations vary from patient to patient. For example, patients
who have nausea and vomiting may need to change their
eating habits. Fried, spicy, or sweet foods may be more
upsetting to your stomach when you feel nauseated.
Cold foods tend to be better tolerated than hot foods.

Some patients develop mouth ulcers, or yeast in the
mouth or throat, during treatment. The presence of
yeast (candidiasis) can affect taste, contributing to loss
of appetite. Report painful sores in the mouth and
throat that limit eating and drinking to your doctor.
Specific medical treatment for the sores as well as

nutritional beverages such as Ensure or Prosure that can help keep you from losing weight during treatment may be recommended.

Some "raw food" diets that are high fiber but low protein are not recommended for cancer patients who need more protein and iron to rebuild their blood counts. Although regular consumption of fruits and vegetables is recommended, patients with very low white blood cell counts may need to avoid raw or uncooked foods because they may still have bacteria in them.

Supplemental vitamins and minerals are not required in a well-balanced diet; however, many patients suffer nausea, poor appetite, or fatigue, which can affect their ability to cook and eat a balanced diet. Although multivitamins and iron supplements do provide essential nutrients, patients under treatment must also consume enough calories and protein. Your doctor may refer you to a dietician if your nutritional needs are not being met and you are losing weight.

Unfortunately, keeping well-nourished and physically healthy does not guarantee that you will avoid a relapse. There are no known modifications of diet that will achieve or prolong remission in brain tumor patients; however, keeping healthy will allow better tolerance of subsequent treatment.

82. Fatigue is a big problem for me. I simply don't have the energy to do anything. What can I do about this?

Fatigue *is* a big problem for cancer patients. In fact, two-thirds of patients report fatigue severe enough to limit their daily activities. Fatigue is not the same as weakness (a loss of strength), but fatigues does involve a sense of generalized weakness, impaired concentration, and tiring easily. Fatigue can be associated with anemia (a low red blood cell count), neutropenia (a low neutrophil count), pain, depression, anxiety, and loss of appetite. Treatment of these factors can sometimes improve the sense of fatigue.

Fatigue can be associated with cancer treatment such as radiation therapy and chemotherapy. The latter can cause anemia and neutropenia. The feeling of fatigue may lessen when the blood count returns to normal. In addition, correcting low blood counts with growth factors such as Procrit (for anemia) and Neupogen (for neutropenia) may allow chemotherapy to continue at the recommended doses.

Cancer patients with normal blood counts may still complain of fatigue. Table 9 lists other causes of fatigue.

Make sure you discuss with your doctor the feeling of fatigue. It is particularly important to note accompanying symptoms such as shortness of breath, constipation, nausea, and muscle weakness, which may have a separate, treatable cause. Strategies for combating fatigue include:

- Participating in aerobic exercise and physical activity
- Keeping a normal sleep/wake cycle
- Planning a rest period following physical exertion
- Setting limits on strenuous work activities
- Conserving energy for specific activities
- Managing stress
- Avoiding foods with high sugar content

Finally, certain vitamin and mineral deficiencies can contribute to fatigue. Supplemental vitamins may be

Table 9   Causes of fatigue in cancer patients

Type of Fatigue	Possible Cause
Cancer-related	Post operative/post-anesthesia Presence of cancer Radiation therapy Chemotherapy
Nutrition-related	Hypoglycemia (low blood sugar) Weight loss Weight gain secondary to steroids
Related to a mood disorder	Depression Anxiety
Related to another illness	Infection/fever Heart disease Lung disease Thyroid disease Chronic pain
Medication-related	Anticonvulsants Pain medication Sedatives Rapid steroid taper

recommended in these cases. However, supplemental vitamins for patients who do not have these deficiencies do not help and could even be harmful.

83. Now that my treatment is over, why am I not happy about it—or at least relieved?

M.L.'s comment:

First, you should keep in mind that your treatments may not end. I thought that because all of the visible tumor was removed during my craniotomy and I had received successfully radiation treatments that my chemotherapy treatments would be "short-lived." After receiving treatments for 12 months I was presented with a number of different options, one of which was to discontinue treatments. After looking at all of the information, my husband and I decided that it would be best for me to continue with my treatments.

Even though I continued with the treatments, I still had many questions such as, "What if my tumor starts to come back even though I stayed on chemo?" or "How long will I have to be on chemo?" and "What will the effects on the rest of my body be if I stay on chemo?" These are tough questions to get answers to because ultimately the decisions must be made by you and your loved ones. The doctors can provide you with some of the answers, but they have to be careful not to tell you what to do. To this day, I still struggle with wanting to know the answer to, "Will I have to take certain medications forever?"

If you aren't happy or relieved when your treatment ends, remember that this is a very common and normal experience. Most people battling brain cancer have a fear of recurrence. This fear is especially difficult to deal with when treatment ends because your healthcare team is no longer surrounding you on a regular basis. There is a natural sense of loss and fear, but you can't allow the fear to take control of your life. Remember, you are in control of your emotions. Part of that control is to be aware of your fears. Don't let your fears dictate the way you live your life.

You have probably realized that you can't control your future, but you can have a positive attitude and live one day at a time. This is a great time to get involved in brain tumor support groups if you haven't already. You can share your fears and emotions with other members of the support group, and there is a very good chance that those same fears and emotions have been felt by other members of the group.

You should also remember that your family and friends are still there for you, even after your treatment ends. Don't be afraid to share your feelings with them and look to them for support and understanding. Also, make sure that you take time to do the things that you enjoy.

All you can do is live one day at a time, but don't be afraid to seek professional help for counseling if you feel that your fears have become excessive.

84. I didn't need physical therapy after my surgery but I've always been physically active. Can I resume regular exercise?

M.L.'s comment:

The answer to this question depends on your particular situation. I would recommend you consult your doctor; however, in my opinion you should strive to begin or resume some sort of exercise as soon as your doctor approves. When I started exercising again I felt that I needed to do it in order to assist in my rehabilitation. I felt like the exercise was helping me to keep up my strength. I remember my doctor telling me that it was good to exercise because it wasn't good to be too sedentary, even in the post-op period. She told me that if patients don't stay active, they are at a higher risk for blood clots in their legs. Another reason why I was eager to start exercising was that the steroids I took contributed to my loss of muscle strength. I was happy to be able to start exercising so I could gain back that strength.

Keep in mind that exercise can be anything from a walk around the block to spending 30 minutes on an exercise bike. When I started exercising again, I didn't try to overdo it. I just wanted to be able to resume some sort of activity. If my doctor told me I could start out with a walk around the block and no more, then that is what I did. As I was able to regain my strength, I gradually was able to increase my level of exercise.

Another bonus is that people who exercise generally feel better mentally as well as physically. I think this is particularly true when someone fears that they have lost strength or coordination after surgery. Working to regain strength and flexibility is an important part of getting well.

85. Will I be allowed to drive?

Driving is clearly a complex task that requires multi-tasking on a level that many adults take for granted. For parents who have had a teenager learning to drive, the anxiety of allowing a sixteen-year-old access to the family car is well understood. Will your teenager anticipate all the hazards on the highway, the stopping distance, and the noise distractions within the car? Insurance companies, of course, know that learning to drive is difficult, which is why rates for young drivers are typically high.

Relearning to drive is no less difficult when a patient has undergone surgery for a brain tumor. Although there may not be apparent motor weakness, visual abnormalities, or blind spots, patients may have slower reaction times and a decreased ability to note subtle environmental clues in traffic. Many neurosurgeons do not allow patients to drive for 6 weeks following surgery. Some neurosurgeons recommend that patients permanently surrender their driver's licenses.

Patients who have suffered seizures, even without loss of consciousness, are restricted from driving. In some states, the patient must be seizure-free for a least one year. The doctor must document that the patient has been counseled regarding driving. Doctors who do allow their brain tumor patients to drive often only recommend drives that are absolutely necessary and involve limited distance, light traffic, and good visibility.

There are rehabilitation programs that perform an assessment of driving using either a simulator or an actual road test under controlled conditions. Reaction time, attention to traffic, judgment of stopping distance, and depth perception are all important facets of relearning to drive.

86. How should I tell my family and friends about my diagnosis?

M.L.'s comment:

Telling someone that you have a brain tumor isn't an easy thing to do, especially to a family member or close friend. In many cases, however, it can be more helpful for you to share your situation with those who care about you the most. They can be there to provide support and also help you to make some of the tough decisions that you'll face. Because there are so many different brain tumor types, I found it necessary to share a great deal of information with my family and friends so that they really understood how serious my illness was. My husband was incredible when it came to this aspect of talking about my situation. He helped me find out as much as possible about brain tumors by gathering information from the doctors as well as the Internet.

My husband, Duane, told my parents about my brain tumor, and then my parents informed the rest of my family. Fortunately, my parents have medical backgrounds, so they could relay the information accurately. If necessary, your doctors and other medical support staff can offer support when you tell your family and friends about your illness. In my case, my parents continued to relay updates to the rest of my family because they all live in Tennessee.

When I was first diagnosed with a brain tumor, my brother, Dennis, and his wife, Kim, came out to see us in Plano, Texas right away. They came before my mother and father did because they were able to leave town right away. Even though I think I was numb for most of the time that they were here (which was only a few day), it was still very comforting to have other family members with me at a time of extreme crisis. My parents came out for my surgery and stayed with me for several weeks. After they left, my sister, Annemarie, came out and stayed with me for almost two weeks.

I remember Duane telling me about how he told our friends Gil and Jayne. Gil's a real tough guy on the outside, but he was very upset. Jayne was really upset and couldn't talk about it without starting to cry, but both of them were there for us no matter how hard it was for them. Gil was great because he always tries to be positive. When appropriate, he would try to interject a little humor somewhere just to keep us laughing. I'll never forget when he came to the hospital wearing black jeans and a black shirt. Duane later told me that Gil had taken a piece of paper and stuck it in his collar so that he appeared to be a priest. It was hard not to laugh at him pretending to be a priest! The

*funny thing was as soon Gil took the fake Roman collar
out, my real pastor arrived at the hospital to see me.*

*In many cases, when I told a friend that I had a brain
tumor I found it easiest to get straight to the point and just
say, "I was recently diagnosed with a brain tumor." Once
they got over the shock of what I said, I found the support
from them to be overwhelming.*

*At one point my husband said he thought that he should
postpone his schooling. I remember telling him that we had
many friends who wanted to help. I didn't think it was
right or fair for him to stop his life if he didn't have to. I
was adamant that he continue with school and he did, but
he would have stopped if I had asked him.*

*I will also say that while so many people were supportive,
there were a few friends who seemed almost uncomfortable
in dealing with my illness and being there for me. At first
this hurt my feelings, but I later learned that this is a common occurrence. There wasn't a thing I could do to change
it. I just came to the realization that dealing with my illness may have reminded those friends of a sad situation
that they may have previously experienced, or that maybe
they just didn't know what to say. I decided to focus on the
fact that I had many more friends who were able to be
there with me, and that's what was important.*

87. How do I tell my young children that I have a brain tumor?

M.L.'s comment:

*Although I don't have children of my own I have several
friends with brain tumors who do have children. I have*

talked to them quite a bit about this subject and have also seen and read information that is intended to be helpful when telling young children that you have a brain tumor. The following comments summarize what I have either been told by others with children or have found to be consistent with information that I have found in other sources.

First of all, always be honest with your children. If your children sense something unusual is happening, then they may use their imagination to create a problem if they aren't told the truth. If that happens what their minds may invent may be much worse than the truth. You'll need to address the children's concerns and talk with them in words that they understand. I have been told that if a brain tumor is described fairly simply to a young child such as, "daddy has a lump in his brain that isn't supposed to be there," that it's easier for them to understand. They need to understand what it means for you to go to the hospital or perhaps have to stay in the hospital for a period of time. Most people that I have spoken to have suggested that a parent needs to answer a child's questions honestly and simply in words that are most appropriate for the child's age. Talking with your children in a loving, truthful, and reassuring manner is essential to their well-being.

Second, be aware of your timing; it's best to talk to your children as soon after your diagnosis as possible. Tell your children as much as you think they need to know in order to calm their fears, but not necessarily everything. In other words, too much information may cause them to worry about things that they can't change. The older the child, the more information you should provide.

Tell your children that you may have treatments that may cause you to lose your hair and make you feel tired. It's OK to tell them that these things are not normal but are part of the process of dealing with a brain tumor. If you're going to have surgery to remove the tumor, you should share this information with them as well. Again, what you say and how you say it will depend on the age of the children. Your children also need to know that having a brain tumor and the signs and symptoms that go with it isn't their fault. Let them know that they can't "catch" your condition by being close to you or touching you.

Don't forget to ask your children if they have any questions. You may be surprised by their concerns, but keep in mind that you also need to be prepared to answer their questions. They may ask you if you're going to die. Your response will depend on the age and maturity of your children. Your specific condition will also be a factor in your response. Once again, you must be truthful with them, but you must always encourage them to be hopeful. Help your children understand that a person who has a brain tumor doesn't necessarily die from it.

A friend of mine told me that she felt it was important to tell her children's teachers. The teachers and school counselors were very supportive and helped her better understand how her children were coping with the situation.

Finally, it's OK if you start to cry when you are telling your children. Crying is a very normal reaction when talking to your children about your situation. Just make sure you tell them why you're crying. It may be because you're sad that you're sick or that you are nervous about some of the changes that may take place as a result of your illness. You should always reassure your children that you'll talk to them about what is happening to you, and that you will do everything you can to make sure that their needs are taken care of by family and friends. Remember to encourage your children to stay positive and to be hopeful.

88. How will treatment of my brain tumor affect my sexuality?

M.L.'s comment:

The answer to this question depends on the person. Some people with brain tumors lose their desire for sex, which can be very normal. There can be a number of causes for this. The location of the brain tumor may be a factor, but because no one has been able to isolate a single area of the brain responsible for the sex drive, the location of your tumor alone can't tell you how your libido will be affected.

Treatments for brain tumors can also have a significant effect on your interest in sex. Whether your treatment involves radiation, chemotherapy, or even the antinausea medication, all of these therapies have direct effects on sexual desire. You can check with your doctor to find out whether any of your treatments have been known to affect libido and how long such effects will last. There are also indirect effects on libido, such as fatigue from radiation or chemotherapy, general weakness, nausea from chemotherapy, and swelling or pain from steroids. Needless to say, when you don't feel good, you may lose interest in sex. However, once your treatments are over, your libido should return.

Depression may also have a negative impact on libido, and having feelings of depression is common for someone who has a brain tumor. In many cases, this is also treatable.

Talk with your doctor to determine the best method to treat your specific situation.

Finally, there may be other factors that may affect your interest in sex. For example, some brain tumor patients may just feel physically unattractive because they may have lost their hair during chemotherapy and radiation (this was the case with me), or perhaps they have gained weight from steroids. Roles within the family may have changed because the patient who used to be the "breadwinner" is now more dependent on other people. All of these factors can be identified and resolved in individual or family therapy; however, the most important thing to remember is that good communication is half the battle.

89. Friends, co-workers, and neighbors who have heard about my brain tumor offer to help, but I'm not sure what I should tell them. What do caregivers and loved ones need to know in order to best support a person with a brain tumor?

M.L.'s comment:

First of all, patients and caregivers need to know that they shouldn't be afraid to ask for help! It's highly likely that you have many family and friends who want to help. Now is the time to let them. Even though my family lived out of town, it seemed as though there wasn't a day that went by that I didn't talk to my mother or father or someone else in my family. Having to be separated by hundreds of miles was hard on all of us, but being able to at least talk on the phone helped me get through some of my toughest days. Some of our closest friends provided not only moral support, but practical help when we needed it the most. For exam-

ple, our dear friends, Gil and Jayne, were tremendously supportive when my parents were here for my surgery. The day of my surgery I had to be at the hospital at 6 a.m., but my surgery wasn't scheduled until around 9 a.m. Duane took me to the hospital that morning, and then around 8 a.m., Gil and Jayne picked up my mother and father and took them to the hospital. Jayne even came by a few days later to take my mother to the salon so that she could get her hair done. The help we received from Gil and Jayne gave my husband more time to be with me. They also helped to relieve some of the stress that comes along with feeling that the caregiver must be responsible for everything.

All of our closest friends continued to be there for not only me, but also for Duane. Gil is one of Duane's best friends, and sometimes I don't know what Duane would have done without having another guy there to just listen and be sympathetic. Many times Gil would give Duane advice on how to deal with some of his fears and concerns about me. He tried to provide as much support as possible.

Duane and I were also able to turn to other close friends such as Bill and Beth. Beth is my dear friend who took me to the emergency room the day I found out that I had a brain tumor. Beth and I have known each other for over 10 years. We used to work together at Nortel Networks. We've been through a lot of ups and downs in each others lives, and we've always been there for each other. She also happens to be married to Bill, whom I got to know while working at Nortel Networks. Beth and Bill have been significant influences in my life and career advancement for the last 5 years. At the time of my diagnosis, Bill was President of eBusiness Solution at Nortel Networks, the division that I was in. One of the greatest things that Bill said was that I didn't need to worry about my responsibilities at work. He told me that I had given Nortel Networks more than 10 years of my life, and now it was time for Nortel Networks to give some of that time back to me. I still don't think that Bill knows how important that statement was to me, even though I've tried to tell him many times. It's difficult to express the peace of mind those words gave. Receiving such support from one of the most senior executives at my company allowed Duane and me to completely focus on the treatments that would help me get better.

As I started to get better, we would have our friends over. Just being able to share good news and bad news with family members or close friends like Bill and Beth or Gil and Jayne provided so much support. Duane and I could tell that it was important to them to understand what we were going through. Our family and friends were there to listen, offer advice, and sometimes to assist us in getting additional information.

PART ELEVEN

Taking Control of Your Future

Are there specific support groups for brain tumor patients? How do I find one?

What records do I need to keep about my treatment? What is the best way to stay organized?

More ...

90. Are there specific support groups for brain tumor patients? How do I find one?

M.L.'s comment:

Yes, there are many good support groups available for brain tumor patients. Some people think that all support groups are the same, but that isn't necessarily true. I have been to a number of different support groups and have found that each of them are as different as the people who are in them. Brain tumor support groups can provide an opportunity to share practical information, offer wisdom, or hear other stories of survival.

I feel very fortunate because my radiation oncologist and his team started a new brain tumor support group at the Baylor/Richardson Cancer Center in Richardson, Texas, and it is the best one that I've ever been associated with. I think what made this one so strong was the level of importance that was placed on this support group not only by my radiation oncologist but also his nurse, Michelle. The Cancer Center and its staff had a reputation for being extremely attentive to its patients. Michelle became more of support person to me than "just a nurse," and she was that way with all of her patients. That level of support carried over into the development of the brain tumor support group that she was instrumental in getting established. I felt like ever time I left one of the sessions that I had just walked out the door with another "nugget" of information that would help me continue to have a positive attitude about myself and my brain tumor. I would strongly recommend that if you're interested in attending a brain tumor support group, you should do so. Support groups can provide tremendous benefit for the patient and the caregiver. Plan to try out a group a few times. If you don't like a particular group, try another one.

There are a number of ways to locate a support group in your area:

- Ask your doctor, nurse, or social worker
- Ask your cancer treatment center or hospital
- Contact the American Brain Tumor Association (see the Appendix for web site information)
- Check your local newspaper or telephone book
- Ask others that you may know with brain cancer.

Keep in mind that if you live in an area that doesn't have a support group for cancer patients, it's still possible to get information and support from brain tumor chat rooms on the Web. This can be a bit tricky, as some people have a tendency to offer medical advice based on their own experience, but it can still be a positive experience for patients and caregivers.

91. What records do I need to keep about my treatment? What is the best way to stay organized?

Although each of your doctors has a record of your treatment, keeping track of what has happened over the course of your treatment is helpful to you, especially if you change doctors or treatment facilities. Some patients write down everything in a calendar, and some patients keep reports in an envelope. Many people have found it convenient to use a loose-leaf notebook with dividers to stay organized. You may want to keep separate sections for pathology reports, laboratory reports, scan reports, notes from clinic visits, and insurance correspondence. Your doctors will usually be happy to give you copies of your reports at your clinic visits. Many patients like to keep a one-page summary in their purse or wallet with their current medications, drug allergies, past medical history, and the names and phone numbers of their doctors. Make sure the summary includes the dates of your operations and radiation therapy, as well as a list of all the chemotherapy drugs you have received. This can be extremely helpful if you have to go to an emergency room when you are away from home.

M.L.'s comment:

I've met a number of people who had impressive record-keeping systems, including bulky binders with color-coded tabs and graphs of everything from white counts to bowel movements! I can certainly see why so much detail is necessary for some patients. Some people may be having a lot of toxicity. By keeping careful records of all the variables involved in their treatment, patients can try to determine what they can change in their treatment to help avoid such toxicity. Fortunately, I didn't have any major problems with toxicity while I was on chemotherapy.

Initially, keeping track of all the medications that I was on was quite a challenge. I found it helpful to keep a list of all of my medication, how often I was to take it, and when I was supposed to take it. This was especially important when I was on chemotherapy because I had to take certain medications in a particular order at a particular time. In addition to listing all of my medications, I also listed the day and date so I could check off when I took my medications for that day. When you're taking as many as 10 to 15 pills per day, this type of timetable can be valuable. By keeping this record, I was assured that I wouldn't miss any of my medications.

One thing that was very helpful was to take my daily planner with me to every appointment. This was great because it had my calendar already in it, along with important names and addresses and extra paper for me to write on. My daily planner also gave me easy access to a list of important questions that I wanted to ask my doctor, and I could write down the answers that my doctors gave me during my visit. For moral support, my husband always went with me to my appointments. If there was something that I missed, he would always remember what was said to me.

I also created a list of my doctors, their telephone numbers, and the names of their nurses or assistants. This became extremely useful when I was receiving radiation treatments because I came in contact with at least six other people in that office (not including my radiation oncologist!) Having my calendar available during radiation treatment helped me keep track of how many weeks I had been receiving radiation therapy and the appointments that I had for MRI scans. I was able to keep track of the dates of when I would be taking chemotherapy. I'd also be able to make a note to remind myself to have my blood taken the week before chemotherapy so that my oncologist could review the results before I started taking any of the drugs.

Having all of this information available right in my calendar made it so much easier for me to communicate information to my doctors. I found that many times the neurosurgeon, radiologist, and oncologist asked me the same questions. Being able to flip to my calendar without having to remember all of the information off the top of my head was invaluable to me.

92. My oncologist told me that even though I'm doing well my tumor will probably come back at some point. He

said, "Hope for the best, but prepare for the worst." I'm hoping for the best, but how do I prepare for the worst?

There are many ways that you can mentally and physically prepare yourself for the possible recurrence of your tumor. Follow up with your doctor regularly for physical examinations and possible re-evaluation by MRI. If your tumor recurs and it can be surgically resected, you should not assume that the second operation will be identical to the first. Some patients heal more slowly following radiation therapy, but some recover sooner because the recurrent tumor was smaller than the original. In some cases, the tumor may change to a different subtype more aggressive than the original tumor. This may require additional treatment after surgery.

If your tumor recurs and cannot be removed, your doctor may refer you to a clinical trial or offer you treatment with radiation therapy or chemotherapy, if you have not already had these treatments.

Patients with a long interval between their original tumor and a recurrent tumor may be surprised to find that a new treatment is available that had not been available previously. Therefore, it is important to discuss with your doctor *at the time of recurrence* how you should be treated.

It is far more difficult to prepare mentally for a recurrent tumor, especially if your treatment options are limited or the recurrent tumor causes severe disability. It is sobering to consider that you may lose the ability to speak or comprehend speech, but some patients do. Finding someone who will make decisions on your behalf and speak for you is critical. A **Durable Power of Attorney for Medical Care (DPA)** allows you to appoint a person who will assume medical decision-making for you if you become disabled. Your DPA should have a thorough understanding of your tumor, your prognosis, and your wishes for further treatment, should you become incapacitated. Remember that your doctor must be able to contact your DPA if you become incapacitated; it is a good idea to give a copy of your DPA document to your doctor with current phone numbers.

Another "worst case scenario" you should consider is the possibility of sudden incapacity that requires life support. Sometimes complications, such as pulmonary embolus, stroke, and seizure require temporary support from ventilators, cardiac resuscitation, and intravenous nutrition. If you do not want to receive life support indefinitely, tell your DPA. You may want to develop an **advanced directive,** a legal document that specifies whether you want specific kinds of supportive care and for how long. Most hospitals now ask patients on admission if they have a DPA for medical care and an advanced directive.

93. I did not have a neuropsychological evaluation before surgery, but my neurologist recommended that I have one now that I have completed radiation therapy. How can neuropsychological tests help me?

M.L.'s comment:

After my surgery, my neurologist suggested that I see a neuropsychologist for testing in order to find out if my surgery

Durable Power of Attorney for Medical Care (DPA)
a legal document that allows a specific family member or other adult to legally make decisions for medical care if the patient becomes incapacitated.

Advanced directives
legal documents that state an individual's preferences for selecting the aggressiveness of supportive care in life-threatening illness.

Taking Control of Your Future

caused any temporary or permanent neurological damage. This evaluation process lasted all day. The tests that were performed went beyond the basic testing that was done when my brain tumor was first discovered. The neuropsychological evaluation primarily consisted of a series of paper-and-pencil question-and-answer tests that are designed to examine various aspects of how the brain functions. My neurologist felt this type of testing was critical in determining whether I would have problems performing common tasks such as balancing my checkbook. The tests would also determine how my short- and long-term memory had been affected by the surgery, if I would be able to return to work, what limitations I may have, and how I would be able to address those limitations.

Some of the tests were very challenging and frustrating at times, but they varied in content and were NOT scored on a pass/fail basis. Therefore, I knew that it was important for me to put forth my best effort on all of the tests.

I was pleasantly surprised when I got the results back. I was expecting the worst, but the results indicated that my memory (verbal and recall) was very good. I was ranked in the 95th percentile! My attention span and capacity had also remained very strong, but the neuropsychologist strongly recommended that I not push myself too hard because fatigue could affect my attention span. This turned out to be true. When I don't take frequent breaks from the computer or when it's late in the afternoon and I've had a fairly busy day with a lot of meetings, my planning and organization skills "slow down" a bit. I'll end up filing something in the wrong folder, or I will forget where I put an important document. Because I'm aware of this potential problem, I try to make sure that I do take frequent breaks from my computer. I also try not to schedule intense or long meetings after about 2 p.m.

I have had a few occasional challenges in the area of "language skills." In general, the test results indicated that my language skills were very good to excellent; however, because my tumor was in my left frontal lobe, the area of the brain where language and memory functions are located, there are times when I search for a particular word and I just can't find it. The neuropsychologist warned me that I might encounter this problem. However, the impact has been minimal. I just get a little frustrated at times. I'm usually the only one who really notices it anyway!

Initially, I wasn't looking forward to the neuropsychological tests (for obvious reasons), but when I look back I'm so glad that I took them. The results have given me so much insight in terms of what to expect with my recovery. If I hadn't taken the tests, I wouldn't have known what problems to expect and, more importantly, how to deal with them. The neuropsychologist was excellent in preparing me for my return to a normal life. I learned that when issues do come up, I shouldn't panic or let my emotions get the best of me. I would strongly recommend a neuropsychological evaluation for all brain tumor patients.

94. How do I discuss prognosis with my doctor?

Prognosis is the expectation of survival related to the presence of a disease. Your doctor relies on knowledge obtained from the medical literature and personal

Prognosis

the long-term outlook for survival and recovery from a disease based upon the patient's current status and the anticipated effect of available treatments.

experience to guide a patient and family through treatment. Doctors are typically reluctant to discuss prognosis until several facts are known: the exact type of tumor, how much of it can be surgically removed, and whether any complications or conditions might impact on treatment.

If you are a newly diagnosed patient, you are probably unfamiliar with many of terms, such as remission, partial remission, response, stable disease, disease progression, and disease-free survival, which doctors used to describe the cancer treatment process. Doctors don't use these terms to avoid discussing cure; they use such terms to more accurately define the probability that the tumor is present, even when it may not cause symptoms or appear on scans. Patients often want to know if they can be cured. The answer to that question is never "no," but it may be "it is unlikely." Even in patients with slow-growing brain tumors, the goal of treatment may be to control the symptoms and prevent neurological disability rather than cure the disease.

The word "cure" is elusive because it is difficult to prove that a tumor will never recur, even after years of remission. There are some tumors that appear to be stable for months or years, only to later grow rapidly into a large mass. For this reason, obtaining scans at regular intervals does not guarantee that a recurrence will be found while the tumor is still very small.

Some patients and their families have been told at the time of diagnosis, "he has two years" or perhaps, "weeks to months." Not surprisingly, a patient's reaction may be disbelief, anger, grief, or fear. Some patients immediately seek a second opinion, hoping to hear a better prognosis. In some cases, this is probably a good idea. The first doctor may have been right, but the timing (immediately after surgery) may have made it difficult for the patient and family to understand and accept the gravity of the situation. A second opinion may help patients accept the situation.

If your doctor informs you that you have a tumor associated with a good prognosis *with treatment*, the prognosis is given with the expectation that you will pursue therapy. For example, patients with primary central nervous system lymphoma can achieve complete remission that can be sustained for years, but the disease is rapidly fatal without treatment.

Your doctor may be reluctant to give you an exact time frame for life expectancy. The type of tumor, its rate of growth, its response to therapy, and the presence or absence of other medical problems may all impact survival. If a doctor gives a range of weeks, months, or years, this range is based on the expected behavior of the tumor, not the possible complications that may occur.

M.L.'s comment:

Two of the most important things that I learned were (1) DON'T be intimidated by your doctors, and (2) ask questions. I have found that most patients and caregivers have many questions and concerns, and they need to get answers to all of them. Your doctors and nurses are the people you should look to for answers. Although the Internet is an incredible resource for information, keep in mind that it's fairly general.

It isn't likely to provide answers to some of your specific questions. Every brain tumor is different. Treatment can be different for each patient. I encourage you to ask your doctors and nurses questions that are specific to you and your situation.

My husband and I had so many questions. Our questions were very specific to the tumor type, at first. Then we wanted to know what (if any) additional treatment would be needed after surgery. We had questions about radiation therapy, chemotherapy, medications, and all of the associated topics within each of those areas. We weren't afraid to ask questions, so we asked every question we had. We felt like we deserved to know the answers. Sometimes I would become frustrated when we would go to a doctor's appointment because my husband would ask so many questions that I couldn't get an opportunity to ask mine. There were a few times when I said, "Hey, do you think you two could be quiet for a minute while I ask a few questions?" Of course, I said it in a joking way.

95. My doctor told me I have a year to live, but I feel fine now. What will happen to me during the next year? How will I die?

While it may be too much to assume that your doctor is correct, for the purpose of this discussion we will assume that he based his opinion on knowing the type of tumor you have and its expected response to treatment. Keep in mind that your tumor could respond much better to treatment, or much worse, than he anticipates; and therefore his estimate of twelve months may be little more than an educated guess.

There are some patients who have very large tumors or multiple tumors at the time of diagnosis. If the tumor cannot be surgically removed safely, the remaining tumor must be successfully treated with another form of therapy if the patient is to survive. Radiation therapy may or may not stop the growth of the tumor. Another form of therapy, such as chemotherapy, may sometimes succeed where radiation failed. However, if the tumor continues to grow through all attempts at treatment, it will ultimately prove fatal.

Patients who have successful surgery to remove the majority of the tumor, called a gross total resection (see Part 4), may still have regrowth of the tumor. This may occur locally (in the same area of the brain as the original tumor), or it may spread to another part of the central nervous system. The ability to control the growth of a new tumor may be limited by the treatment of the original tumor. Further radiation may not be possible, or the patient may have developed a resistance to chemotherapy. The symptoms caused by an enlarging tumor may be slowly progressive, such as the gradual onset of weakness and poor coordination. Sometimes patients with enlarging tumors have a more rapid onset of weakness, confusion, or imbalance. In a few instances, the sudden change may be related to bleeding within the tumor.

Patients with all types of cancer may become more vulnerable to complications such as infection, blood clots, and malnutrition. In addition, patients with primary or metastatic brain tumors may suffer seizures, headaches, vomiting, and difficulty swallowing. These conditions may bring on new problems that result in even further disability. A patient who has difficulty swallowing, for example, may choke on food or fluids, which can lead to pneumonia. Pneumonia may cause shortness of breath, fever, and loss of appetite. A patient who feels short of breath is unlikely to have enough energy to keep physically active, but the lack of activity may increase the risk of blood clots in the vessels of the legs. Swelling and pain in the legs may also limit physical activity, confining the patient to bed. Unfortunately, these complications may require frequent hospital or emergency room visits. It may be difficult to anticipate and prevent these complications or to reverse many of these conditions once they occur. It is estimated that 70% of cancer patients die of complications, such as infection, rather than the cancer directly.

No one likes to think about such complications when feeling well, but it is helpful nonetheless to talk frankly with one's doctor about the possibility of becoming progressively disabled. The patient and doctor can agree on a hospital that will be used, if necessary, and a nursing service that can provide care at home. It is also important to discuss with family members the aggressiveness of supportive care desired. Advanced directives (see Question 92) are instructions to doctors and caregivers specifying whether life support equipment, artificial nutrition, and other supportive measures should be used if you become too disabled to direct your further care.

96. My neurosurgeon, radiation oncologist, neurologist, and medical oncologist don't always agree. Who is in charge?

The answer might surprise you: *you* are in charge. Although your doctors may have several years of experience in their respective specialties, it is still up to you to weigh their recommendations. If your doctors are giving you conflicting answers, make sure you find out why.

A common area of disagreement among doctors is in regard to the frequency of follow-up MRI scans. Your neurosurgeon may suggest that you have scans done at three-month intervals. Your oncologist, on the other hand, may recommend that you have scans done after a specific number of cycles of chemotherapy. Some drugs, such as BCNU and CCNU, are given every 6 to 8 weeks. Other drugs, such as Temodar, are given in 4-week cycles. Your oncologist may change the time between scans to coincide with your chemotherapy cycles. Keep in mind that your doctors may differ in their recommendations for appropriate follow-up, so you may need to remind one doctor of the follow-up procedures your other doctor has already scheduled. For example, if you don't remind your radiation oncologist that your neurologist has already ordered an MRI, you could be scheduled for MRIs on different days at different facilities!

Another area of vital importance is your medication profile. Although all of your doctors want and need a current medication profile, it is up to you to know exactly which medications you are taking. You are also responsible for making sure that you have enough refills. If you are taking anticonvulsant medication, your neurologist may ask for blood tests to check the level of the drug. If you are also taking chemotherapy, you may be able to arrange for these blood tests to be done when the laboratory tests for your oncologist are done. If you make sure all of your doctors are aware of the laboratory tests you need, you might be able to save yourself some time—and a needle stick, too.

Some specialists keep their colleagues informed of a patient's progress through letters and phone calls. Others depend on the patient to relay information to the other doctors involved in his or her care. If you find that one of your doctors seems to be unaware of recommendations that another doctor has made, bring this to the doctor's attention immediately. It may be a simple matter of a delay in the transcription and mailing of dictated letters or notes. By keeping copies of your scan reports and laboratory tests, you can update any of your doctors who are temporarily "out of the loop."

97. My doctor told me that my treatment is not working and that I should consider hospice. If I choose hospice, isn't that just giving up?

Hospice services vary in different communities, but in general, hospice allows patients to receive care for the symptoms of their disease when treatment options to cure or control the disease are unavailable or no longer effective. For example, a woman who has a recurrent brain tumor has undergone surgery, radiation therapy, and chemotherapy. During her last chemotherapy cycle she had frequent complications requiring hospitalization. This particular patient may not benefit from additional therapy because her quality of life has been compromised by complications. If there are no further treatment alternatives that are likely to be of benefit, or if all treatment options appear to be equally toxic, she may be offered hospice.

Hospice services provide care for patients in the home or hospital setting. Hospice nurses work closely with doctors so that symptoms such as seizures, headache, fever, shortness of breath, and pain are controlled with medications or other interventions. Hospice services may be paid for by government programs or by private insurance. Some communities have hospice services available for indigent patients.

Do not think of hospice services as giving up an opportunity for effective treatment. Doctors typically do not refer their patients to hospice care if further treatment is likely to succeed. Acceptance of this prognosis is an important requirement for patients entering hospice.

Hospices commonly have social workers, counselors, and chaplains available to help patients discuss financial concerns and end-of-life decisions. Patients and hospice workers often develop close friendships because of their frequent contact. This relationship can be a great comfort to many patients. Hospice workers also work with surviving family members following the death of the patient to help them cope with the loss.

Remember that hospice workers are trained to alleviate symptoms. They do not do anything to hasten death. However, the use of intravenous fluids, intravenous antibiotics, and artificial feedings is generally discouraged in terminally ill patients because these measures do not ease suffering.

Taking Control of Your Future

98. I was told that my tumor is rare, and it has been difficult to find information about it. How can I find out more about my tumor?

Trying to find information about any kind of brain tumor can be a daunting task. The Internet has simplified the process greatly. People who were diagnosed with a brain tumor just 10 or 15 years ago did not have this valuable resource available to them. Web resources, such as Yahoo, AltaVista, and Google, offer easy-to-use search tools that will lead you to numerous Web pages focusing specifically on brain tumors. Of course, you can always consult your local library or the medical library at your local hospital or university, but by far the fastest way to find information is via the Internet.

When researching your tumor, you must know the exact name of it. You can find the tumor name in your pathology report. For example, it is not enough to know that you have a pineal tumor. Your tumor may be a pineocytoma, a pineoblastoma, a germ cell tumor, or another type. If your pathology report uses a modifier such as "anaplastic," "malignant," or "metastatic," you must include these terms in your search.

If you enter the term "central neurocytoma" into the search engine at *www.google.com*, the site retrieves 739 references. You can refine these search results by adding other key words or phrases. In this example, adding "surgical resection" to the search terms, and modifying the search results to include only Web pages in English that have been updated in the past six months drops your search results down to a more manageable 49 references.

Many of the web pages in your search results will be neuropathology, neurosurgery, or other medical Web sites. However, there are patient resources also available. Neurosurgery://On-Call (*www.neurosurgery.org/health/patient/detail.asp?DisorderID=79*) is provided by the American Association of Neurological Surgeons and Congress of Neurological Surgeons. This review of brain tumors contains a paragraph describing the location of central neurocytomas, the age range of patients, and an explanation of treatment options.

Finding more detailed information about central neurocytomas is also possible through medical databases such as Medline or Cancerlit. But if you are interested in a broad discussion of the treatment of central neurocytoma (surgical resection, radiation therapy, and long-term prognosis), you should consider limiting your search to review articles. For most medical literature, only a short summary of the article (the abstract) is available online, but the entire article can be obtained from a medical library.

99. Why has there been so little progress in fighting brain tumors?

Brain tumors are relatively uncommon, especially when they are compared with lung cancer, breast cancer, and prostate cancer. These "big three" cancers are responsible for 44% of all cancers diagnosed in the United States. Brain tumors constitute less than 2% of the total number of cancers diagnosed. Because of effective screening, breast and prostate cancers are often diagnosed at earlier stages, and less than 20% of patients die of their disease. In contrast, 77% of brain tumor patients

Taking Control of Your Future

will die of their tumor or complications related to their tumor. There are no effective screening strategies for the common adult brain tumor, glioblastoma multiforme, and even "early" diagnosis of a small, resectable tumor may not associated with a favorable prognosis.

The many different subtypes of brain tumors require different treatment strategies. Ideally, new treatment approaches would be developed in a clinical trial that monitors all patients for response to therapy and the toxicity of treatment. However, only about 4% of all cancer patients are enrolled in clinical trials. Even the most promising new therapy must be rigorously tested before it can be offered to all patients, but if few patients participate in clinical trials, new therapies cannot become the standard of care.

Assuming that a new drug has been well studied in clinical trials, there are often other hurdles that limit access to the drug. For example, drugs that have been FDA-approved for one type of tumor may be considered off label for the treatment of brain tumors, and some insurers will not cover the cost of the drug in these cases. Patients who cannot find a way to support the high cost of the drug lose out on a possible treatment option.

Brain tumor patients also have traditionally had less exposure in the media. Celebrities who have been diagnosed and treated for a brain tumor rarely make public statements concerning the need for further research funding. Although some brain tumor survivors have neurological deficits that prevent them from working, thousands of others work full time, raise families, and contribute to their communities. Despite these achievements, there has yet to be any national recognition of the efforts of brain tumor survivors.

Brain tumor patients and their families and friends can do much to promote public education about brain tumors. Encouraging financial support for brain tumor research, participating in national brain tumor advocacy groups, and keeping up with brain tumor information by visiting web sites such as *www.virtualtrials.com* are all ways to further brain tumor research and education.

How to Survive a Brain Tumor

1. Know your enemy. The more you know about your enemy's strengths and weaknesses, the better you can fight it.

2. Know your strengths. Keep healthy and fit.

3. Know your weaknesses. If there's something that you can improve, do it. If you can't change it, accept it and move on.

4. Know your allies. If you don't think your doctor is 100% dedicated to the battle, you may need to find another one.

5. Know your weapons. Some treatments for brain tumors sound pretty scary (and pretty toxic), but if they work against the enemy, they're what you need.

6. Maintain your arsenal. Don't run out of the medications you need. Don't let your insurance lapse; if it does, look for as many different funding resources you can.

7. Find some comrades in arms. No one else really knows what it's like to be in the trenches, and some of your best friends could be made on the battlefield.

8. Take time for rest and relaxation. You need it to keep fighting.

9. Remember that an army moves on its stomach. If you don't get adequate nutrition, you'll be defeated.

Taking Control of Your Future

10. Look to experienced leaders in your treatment team for guidance. Respect them, work with them, and remember your common objective.

11. Check your position from time to time. Those follow-up appointments, labs, and MRIs keep the enemy under scrutiny.

12. Don't be afraid to use whatever weapons are available. Unconventional weaponry (such as clinical trials) can surprise the enemy.

13. Anticipate occasional setbacks. Keep mentally prepared to engage more vigorously with the enemy if necessary.

14. Don't ignore warnings from your body. Fever, pain, and shortness of breath require immediate attention!

15. Scout for locations of refuge if you ever need one. Hospitals that are ill-equipped to deal with your enemy aren't good places to be.

16. Keep the folks back home informed about how the battle is going.

17. Be patient with others who don't know the enemy as well as you do. They have other battles to fight.

18. Kiss your sweetheart as often as possible and always with the thought that it could be the last.

19. Pray for your comrades, your family, and yourself. Pray for you to have courage, and then act as though your prayer was already answered.

20. Remember that the enemy can take your life, but not your spirit. Make sure that you spread your spirit around to so many places that the enemy can never destroy it.

100. *Where can I go for further information?*

Many hospitals and cancer centers have patient libraries and resource centers with booklets and reading lists about specific topics. The National Cancer Institute and National Institutes of Health publish a wide variety of books about clinical trials, cancer diagnosis and treatment, and nutritional support for cancer patients. Booklets are available free of charge by calling 1–800–4—CANCER and can be viewed online at *www.cancer.gov.*

Organizations

National Organizations for Brain Tumor Patients

American Brain Tumor Association
2720 River Road, Suite 146
Des Plaines, Illinois 60018
Phone: 847–827–9910
www.abta.org
Provides information free of charge about brain tumors, and sponsors research
   grants and regional "Town Hall Meetings." The gray ribbon "Brain Tumor
   Awareness" lapel pin is available from the ABTA store.

National Brain Tumor Foundation
414 Thirteenth Street, Suite 700
Oakland, California 94612
Phone: 510–839–9777
Web site: www.braintumor.org
A non-profit organization which sponsors several community Angel Adven-
   tures, which raise funds for brain tumor research and provide an opportunity
   for brain tumor patients and families to participate in a walk together.

The Brain Tumor Society
124 Watertown Street, Suite 3H
Watertown, Massachusetts 02472–2500
Phone: 800–770–8287
Web site: www.tbts.org
A web site that includes information about events and conferences, including
   teleconferences and live web casts. An extensive book list about brain tumors
   and brain tumor survivors is available by request and online.

Pediatric Brain Tumor Foundation of the U.S.
315 Ridgefield Court
Asheville, North Carolina 28806
Phone: 800–253–6530
Web site: www.pbtfus.org
Promotes public awareness of pediatric brain tumors and raises
 money in support of adult and pediatric brain tumor research.

Brain Tumor Foundation for Children, Inc.
1835 Savoy Drive, Suite 316
Atlanta, Georgia 30341
Phone: 770–458–5554
Web site: www.btfcgainc.org
A nonprofit organization to promote awareness and support
 research for children with brain tumors.

Candlelighters Childhood Cancer Foundation
7910 Woodmont Avenue, Suite 460
Bethesda, Maryland 20814
Phone: 800–366–2223
Web site: www.candlelighters.org
A resource for families of children with cancer.

Other Useful Resources and Web Sites

National Center for Complementary and Alternative Medicine
P.O. Box 8218
Silver Spring, Maryland 20907
Phone: 301–435–5042
Web site: www.nccam.nih.gov
This site contains information about complementary and alterna-
 tive medicine, including current clinical trials using these
 methods.

American Cancer Society
1599 Clifton Road, NE
Atlanta, Georgia 30329
Phone: 800–ACS–2345
Web site: www.CANCER.org
This is a web site that is easy to use and has information on a
 wide variety of topics, including chemotherapy and radiation
 therapy.

Musella Foundation for Brain Tumor Research and Information

Web site: www.virtualtrials.com

This is a fantastic resource for anyone newly diagnosed with a brain tumor, anyone starting chemotherapy or radiation therapy, or someone who's looking for a clinical trial. It is well organized, regularly updated and may be the only brain tumor resource you'll ever need. It also has links to many other useful sites.

NeedyMeds

Web site: www.NeedyMeds.com

If you can't afford your medication, this site can give you some useful resources, sometimes free from the manufacturer.

Oncolink

Web site: www.Oncolink.com

This site, sponsored by the Abramson Cancer Center of the University of Pennsylvania, contains information on a wide variety of cancer topics, including clinical trials.

Vital Options International

Web site: www.vitaloptions.org

An international organization for young adults with cancer, hosting a weekly syndicated radio show and web cast on a variety of topics.

CancerCare

Web site: www.cancercare.org

CancerCare is a nonprofit organization providing free professional help to patients with all types of cancers. This web site includes information for financial assistance, support groups, cancer and sexuality, and many other topics.

CancerSource.com

Web site: www.CancerSource.com

This is a well-illustrated and comprehensive resource for cancer patients and families about diagnosis and treatment options, including more advanced topics for nursing and medical professionals. This site allows you to receive a personalized e-mail newsletter. It is partnered with Jones and Bartlett Publishers, allowing purchase of books on-line.

Selected United States Cancer Centers with Brain Tumor Programs

Children's National Medical Center
Washington, D.C.
Phone: 202–884–2120
Web site: www.cnmc.org

University of Alabama at Birmingham
Birmingham, Alabama
Web site: www.braintumor.uab.edu

Cedars-Sinai Maxine Dunitz Neurosurgical Institute
Los Angeles, California
Phone: 310–423–7900
Web site: www.cedars-sinai.edu/mdsni

UCLA Medical Center
Los Angeles, California
Phone: 310–825–5074
Web site: www.neurooncology.ucla.edu

University of Southern California
Los Angeles, California
Phone: 323–226–7421
Web site: www.usc.edu/medicine/neurosurgery

University of California at San Francisco
San Francisco, California
Phone: 415–353–2966
Web site: www.ucsf.edu.nabtc.org

University of Colorado Health Sciences Center
Aurora, Colorado
Phone: 720–848–0116
Web site: www.uch.uchs.edu/uccc/patient/neuroonc.html

H. Lee Moffitt Cancer Center and Research Institute
Tampa, Florida
Phone: 813–632–1730
Web site: www.moffitt.usf.efu/clinical/nonc/index.htm

Brigham & Women's Hospital
Boston, Massachusetts
Phone: 617–732–6810
Web site: www.boston-neurosurg.org

Massachusetts General Hospital
Boston, Massachusetts
Phone: 617–726–7851
Web site: www.brain.mgh.harvard.edu

Johns Hopkins Hospital
Baltimore, Maryland
Phone: 410–955–0703
Web site: www.nabtt.org/johns.html

National Cancer Institute
Bethesda, Maryland
Phone: 301–402–6298
Web site: www.dcs.nci.nih.gov/trials

Henry Ford Hospital
Detroit, Michigan
Phone: 313–916–1340
Web site: www.nabtt.org/henry.html

University of North Carolina–Lineburger Comprehensive Cancer Center
Chapel Hill, North Carolina
Phone: 919–966–1374
Web site: www.cancer.med.unc.edu

Duke University Medical Center
Durham, North Carolina
919–684–5301
Web site: www.cancer.duke.edu/btc

Dartmouth-Hitchcock Medical Center
Lebanon, New Hampshire
Phone: 603–650–6312
Web site: www.dartmouth.edu/dms/nccc/brain.htm

Memorial Sloan-Kettering Cancer Center
New York, New York
Phone: 800–525–2225
Web site: www.mskcc.org

New York Presbyterian Hospital
Weill Cornell Medical Center
New York, New York
Phone: 212–746–2438

Children's Hospital of Philadelphia
Philadelphia, Pennsylvania
Phone: 215–590–3129
Web site: www.chop.edu

Children's Hospital of Pittsburgh
Pittsburgh, Pennsylvania
Phone: 412–692–5881
Web site: www.neurosurgery.pitt.edu

St. Jude Children's Research Hospital
Memphis, Tennessee
Phone: 901–495–3604
Web site: www.stjude.org/brain

Presbyterian Hospital of Dallas
Dallas, Texas
Phone: 214–345–4200
Web site: www.phscare.org

M.D. Anderson Cancer Center
Houston, Texas
Phone: 713–794–1285
Web site: www.mdanderson.org

University of Utah/Huntsman Cancer Institute
Salt Lake City, Utah
Phone: 801–581–6908
Web site: www.hci.utah.edu/5065.html

University of Wisconsin Medical School
Madison, Wisconsin
Phone: 608–263–5009
Web site: www.humonc.wisc.edu

Fox Chase Cancer Center
Philadelphia, Pennsylvania
Phone: 215–717–3005
Web site: www.neuro-oncology.org

Other Helpful Organizations

American Institute for Cancer Research
1759 R Street NW
Washington, DC 20009
Phone: 800–843–8114 or 202–328–7744
Web site: www.aicr.org

Americans with Disabilities Act
U.S. Dept. of Justice
950 Pennsylvania Avenue
Washington, DC 20530
Phone: 800–514–0301
Web site: www.usdoj.gov/crt/ada/adahom1.htm

National Coalition for Cancer Survivorship
1010 Wayne Avenue, Suite 505
Silver Spring, Maryland 20910
Phone: 877–NCCSYES (622–7937)
Web site: www.cansearch.org
Acts as a clearinghouse and helps cancer survivors, their families,
and friends find local support groups, learn health insurance
options, and prevent employment bias.

Appendix

National Family Caregivers Association
10400 Connecticut Avenue, #500
Kensington, Maryland 20895
Phone: 800–896–3650
Web site: www.nfcacares.org
Provides education, support, respite care and advocacy for caregivers. Their toll-free information line provides referrals to
   caregiver support groups as well as information on how to start
   a caregivers' support group.

National Hospice Organization
Phone: 800–658–8898
Web site: www.nho.org
Promotes quality care for the terminally ill and their families.
   Their help line refers callers to local hospices, and they can also
   inform callers as to whether a facility is licensed and Medicare
   certified.

Patient Advocate Foundation
739 Thimble Shoals Boulevard, Suite 704
Newport News, VA 23606
Phone: 800–532–5274
Web site: www.patientadvocate.org

Glossary

Abstract: Brief summary of a scientific paper.

Advanced directives: Legal documents that state an individual's preferences for selecting the aggressiveness of supportive care in life-threatening illness.

Alopecia: Hair loss.

Alternative therapy: Treatment used in lieu of standard medical therapies.

Anemia: Low red blood cell count; may cause tiredness, weakness, and shortness of breath.

Animal models: Laboratory animals that have diseases similar to those in humans.

Anti-angiogenesis: Property of a drug or other treatment that prevents the formation of new blood vessels.

Antiemetic medications: Drugs that prevent nausea and vomiting.

Astrocytes: One of the major types of glial cells of the nervous system.

Astrocytoma: A glioma that has developed from astrocytes.

Benign: Not cancerous; not life-threatening.

Bioavailability: Chemical property of a drug describing its absorption through the gastrointestinal tract when taken orally.

Biopsy: Surgical removal of a small piece of tissue or a tumor for microscopic examination.

Blood-brain barrier: Tightly joined cells in the blood vessels of the brain that prevent the ready diffusion of substances into the brain tissue.

Bone marrow reserve: Term used by oncologists to describe the expectation of recovery of bone marrow cells following treatment with chemotherapy or radiation therapy.

Boost: High dose of fractionated radiation.

Brachytherapy: Internal radiation therapy that involves placing radioactive material near or in the tumor.

Brain stem: That part of the CNS responsible for a number of "unconscious" activities, including breathing, heart rate, wakefulness and sleep.

Cancerous: Abnormal and uncontrolled growth of cells in the body that may spread, injure areas of the body and lead to death.

Centigray (cGy): Unit of radiation, equal to one rad.

CNS (central nervous system): Pertaining to the brain and spinal cord.

Cerebellum: Part of the brain located at the back of the head, under the cerebrum and in front of the brain stem. Controls balance and coordination, affecting movements of the same side of the body.

Cerebrum: The largest area of the brain; divided into the right and left cerebral hemispheres.

Chemotherapy: The use of chemical agents (drugs) to treat cancer

Choroid plexus: Two spongelike tissues in the lateral ventricles that produce the spinal fluid.

Clinical trial: A research protocol that is designed to answer a question regarding a population of patients with disease or who are at risk for disease.

Cobalt: A radioactive isotope used in the treatment of cancer.

Complementary treatment: Treatment used in conjunction with standard treatment for disease.

Complete remission (CR): The complete resolution of all signs and symptoms of disease.

Conformal radiation therapy: Three-dimensional radiation using images from CT and MRI to plan precise fields of radiation that may be contoured around structures such as the eyes or the brainstem.

Conventional radiation: The type of radiation therapy delivered by a linear accelerator, usually divided over several treatments.

Coronal image: Image that divides the brain into front (anterior) and back (posterior) and shows best the deeper and more central areas of the brain.

Corpus callosum: A prominent nerve fiber bundle in the center of the brain connecting the cerebral hemispheres.

Cortex: The outer surface of the cerebral hemispheres; often called the gray matter.

Corticosteroid: A naturally occurring hormone produced by the adrenal cortex, or a synthetic hormone having similar properties; often used to treat edema (swelling) in leaky capillaries of the brain.

Cranial nerves: Nerves that arise from the base of the brain or the brainstem that provide sensory and motor function to the eyes, nose, ears, tongue, and face.

Craniotomy: A surgical "cutting" of an opening into the skull.

Computed Tomography (CT scan): Computerized series of x-rays that create a detailed cross-sectional image of the body.

Deep vein thrombosis (DVT): Blood clot forming in deep veins, often with impaired or sluggish blood flow.

DNA (deoxyribonucleic acid): The genetic information in the cell nucleus, containing directions on cell growth, division, and function.

Dominant: Ruling or controlling. The cerebral hemisphere that controls speech formation is referred to as the dominant hemisphere.

Durable Power of Attorney for Medical Care (DPA): A legal document that allows a specific family member or other adult to legally make decisions for medical care if the patient becomes incapacitated.

Edema: Swelling or fluid build-up.

Electroencephalogram (EEG): A recording of the electrical impulses of the brain using electrodes attached to the scalp.

Ependymal: One of the major types of glial cells, which line the surfaces of the ventricles of the brain and the center canal of the spinal cord.

Ependymoma: Tumor that has developed from abnormal ependymal cells.

Exclusion criteria: Characteristics specified in a clinical trial that render the patient ineligible for the study.

External beam radiation: The type of radiation therapy delivered by a linear accelerator.

Fields: The volume of tissue to be treated during radiation therapy.

Fissures: The deep folds that separate each cerebral hemisphere into lobes.

Food and Drug Administration (FDA): A federal institution charged with approving and regulating medications, foodstuff, and other products for human consumption.

Foramen magnum: A large hole at the base of the skull; it serves as the boundary between the brain stem and the spinal cord.

Fourth ventricle: One of the spinal fluid pathways in the midline of the brain, between the brainstem and the cerebellum.

Fraction: Single treatment of radiation.

Frontal lobe: The anterior (toward the face) area in the cerebral hemisphere involved in emotion, thought, reasoning, and behavior.

Functional MRI: A type of MRI that detects the changes in red blood cells and capillaries as they deliver oxygen to "functioning" parts of the brain.

Gamma Knife: Type of stereotactic radiation designed to deliver radiation from multiple cobalt sources, computer-focused to a small area or multiple small areas.

Generalized seizure: Seizure involving both hemispheres of the brain.

Glial: Supportive tissue of the brain, includes astrocytes, oligodendrocytes, and ependymal cells. Unlike neurons, they do not conduct electrical impulses and can reproduce.

Grade: Term used to describe the degree to which tumor tissue resembles normal tissue under the microscope.

Gray (Gy): Modern unit of radiation dosage.

Gross total resection: Removal of all visible portions of a tumor.

Hemisphere: One of the two halves of the cerebrum or the cerebellum.

High grade: Tumor that has a rapid growth rate; the cells may appear disorganized and distorted.

Image-guided surgery: *see* neuronavigation

Informed Consent: Process of explaining to the patient all risks and complications of a procedure or treatment before it is done. Informed consents are signed by the patient, a parent of a minor child, or a legal representative.

Intermediate grade: Tumors that have features of aggressiveness and growth characteristics between low- and high-grade tumors.

Interstitial brachytherapy: Radiation therapy that is administered from the inside of the tumor cavity, with a source of radiation therapy such as radioactive iodine or iridium.

Intra-arterial administration: Injection into an artery that supplies blood to the tumor.

Intrathecal administration: The injection of a drug directly into the spinal fluid.

Intracavitary administration: The administration of a drug directly into the tumor cavity.

Intra-operative MRI: An "MRI guidance" system available in operating rooms designed to function with an MRI scanner.

Intra-operative radiation: A dose of radiation given directly to the tumor site immediately after the surgery to remove the tumor.

Investigators: Physicians or other individuals who are involved with an experimental study or clinical trial.

Ionizing radiation: A form of energy that knocks electrons out of their normal orbits.

Lateral ventricles: The two elongated, curved openings in each cerebral hemisphere connecting with two slit-like openings in the center of the brain.

Leptomeningeal metastases: The spread of cancer cells through the spinal fluid, producing a coating around the brain or spinal cord.

Linear accelerator: A machine used in radiation therapy that is able to create man-made ionizing radiation in the form of x-rays to penetrate through tissue into a tumor.

Local radiation therapy: Radiation to a specific area rather than to the entire brain.

Localizing: Symptoms suggesting that a specific area of the nervous system is involved; for example, speech disturbance, weakness of one side of the body, or loss of vision.

Low grade: Tumors that have few cells dividing at any one time, often resembling normal tissue.

Lumbar puncture: Method of obtaining a sampling of spinal fluid from the space between the lumbar vertebrae.

Lymphocytes: Type of white blood cell found in lymphatic tissue such as lymph nodes, spleen, and bone marrow.

Magnetic resonance imaging (MRI): A radiographic study based on the acquisition of anatomical information using resonance from atoms in a strong magnetic field.

Magnetic Resonance Spectroscopy (MRS): A study similar to conventional MRI that measures chemical compounds within the brain.

Malignant: Cancerous; cells that exhibit rapid, uncontrolled growth.

Malignant transformation: The development of more destructive, invasive, or rapid growth in a previously benign or indolent tumor.

Margin: An area around the edge of a tumor visualized on brain scan, which may include scattered tumor cells.

Medical history: A detailed accounting by the patient that helps a physician to determine the length and severity of an illness as well as previous personal and family health history.

Medical oncologist: A physician who performs comprehensive management of cancer patients throughout all phases of care; specializes in treating cancer with medicine.

Meningeal carcinomatosis: *See* Leptomeningeal spread.

Meninges: Membranes covering the brain and spinal cord, consisting of the pia, arachnoid, and dura.

Metabolism: The normal physical and chemical changes within living tissue.

Metastasis: The spread of cancer from the initial cancer site to other parts of the body through the lymphatic system, the bloodstream, or the spinal fluid.

Metastatic tumors: Cancer that has spread outside of the organ or structure in which it arose to another area of the body.

Mini-Mental Status Examination: A brief verbal and written examination that tests orientation, memory, calculation, language, and figure drawing on a 30-point scale.

Monocytes: Type of white blood cells normally found in the lymph nodes, spleen, bone marrow, and within tissue.

Multifocal: Having more than one point of origin.

Negative margin: A phrase used when normal tissue is found at the edge of the biopsy sample.

Neurological deficit: Partial or complete loss of muscle strength, sensation, or other brain functions; may be temporary or permanent.

Neurological examination: Part of the physical examination testing general intellectual function, speech, motor function, memory, sensation, reflexes, and cranial nerve functions.

Neuronavigation: Pre-operative or intra-operative imaging information which allows the surgeon to view images in the operating room during surgery to localize normal brain structures and tumor.

Neuropathologist: Pathologist specializing in the diagnosis of diseases of the peripheral and central nervous system.

Neuropsychologist: Professionals who specialize in the effect of brain injury on behavior and cognition. They help identify ways to improve relearning and to compensate for neurological functions that are impaired.

Neuroradiologist: Physician trained to interpret x-rays, CT scans, and other radiological images of the brain.

Neuron: Nerve cell that conducts electrical or chemical signals.

Neurosurgeon: Surgeon specializing in the diagnosis and treatment of disease of the central and peripheral nervous system, including the skull, spine, and blood vessels.

Neutropenia: A lower than normal neutrophil count.

Neutrophil: Type of white blood cell.

Noncancerous: Tissue that does not appear to be malignant; may be benign or normal.

Nondiagnostic: A tissue sample that does not contain adequate information for determining the presence or absence of disease.

Nonlocalizing: Symptoms not confined, limited, or contained to a specific area; may be attributed to other illnesses, depression, or stress. Examples include fatigue, lack of concentration, or nausea.

Occipital lobe: Area in the cerebral hemispheres that interpret visual images as well as the meaning of written words.

Occupational therapy: Assists patients in normalizing activities of daily living, such as bathing, brushing teeth, cutting meat, and dressing.

Off-label drug: A drug that is approved by the FDA for one type of treatment but may be prescribed for other conditions.

Oligodendrocytes: One of the major types of glial cells.

Oligodendroglioma: Abnormal oligodendrocytes that grow into a tumor.

Ommaya reservoir: A hollow, slightly dome-shaped device is attached to a catheter that is surgically implanted into the cerebral ventricle. Chemotherapy is administered by injection into the reservoir and catheter.

Open biopsy: Procedure allowing a neurosurgeon to directly visualize the surface of the brain prior to removal of a piece of a tumor.

Parietal lobe: Area in the cerebral hemispheres that controls sensory and motor information.

Partial remission (PR): Shrinkage or partial disappearance of tumor, but with evidence that some of the tumor still exists.

Partial resection: Procedure that allows a neurosurgeon to directly visualize the surface of the brain prior to removal of some, but not all, of a tumor.

Partial seizure: Seizure involving only one area or lobe of the brain.

Pathologist: A physician trained to examine and evaluate cells, tissue, and organs for the presence of disease.

Pathology report: Summary of the gross (specimen visible to the naked eye) and microscopic analysis of tissue and/or fluid removed during surgery.

Positron Emission Tomography (PET): A nuclear medicine imaging test that detects differences in metabolism; often used to differentiate between healthy and abnormal tissue.

Pharmacokinetics: Study of how the body breaks down a drug after it is administered.

Phase I trial: Study of a small group of patients to determine effectiveness and the side effects of a new treatment.

Phase II trial: Study of a group of similar patients to determine whether there is a statistical likelihood that a new treatment will be effective against a tumor.

Phase III trial: Compares two or more kinds of treatment in two or more similar groups of patients, with one group of patients receiving the standard, or control, therapy.

Physiatrist: Physician who specializes in physical medicine and rehabilitation and in prescribing the components of a rehabilitation program.

Physical therapy: Therapy aimed at recovery from weakness, loss of coordination, or limited endurance.

Pilot study: Small study designed to test an idea or treatment prior to a larger clinical trial; also called *feasibility study*.

Placebo: A medication ("sugar pill") or treatment that has no effect on the body, often used in experimental studies to determine if the experimental medication/treatment has an effect.

Positive margin: A phrase used when cancer cells are found at the edge of the biopsy sample.

Preclinical study: Study that uses live animals or cell cultures to determine the effectiveness and toxicity of a treatment.

Primary brain tumor: Tumors that develop from mutations of normal cells that originate in the brain, the spinal cord, or the meninges.

Prognosis: The long-term outlook for survival and recovery from a disease based upon the patient's current status and the anticipated effect of available treatments.

Proliferation index: A measurement of the growth and division rate of cells obtained from a biopsy specimen, using special stains.

Protocol: A research plan for how a therapy is given and to whom it is given.

Pulmonary embolus: Blood clot that travels through the veins and the heart, eventually occluding one or more pulmonary arteries.

Radiation necrosis: An area of injured normal glial cells and blood vessels that may occur several months after radiation therapy.

Radiation oncologist: A physician who specializes in treating cancer with radiation.

Radiation physicist: A scientist trained to determine the dose and accuracy of radiation therapy equipment.

Radiation therapy: Treatment that uses high-dose x-rays or other high energy rays to kill cancer cells and shrink tumors.

Radiosensitivity: A tumor's susceptibility to growth inhibition or cell killing by radiation therapy.

Radiosignal: In MRI, the image produced by resonance of hydrogen atoms in a magnetic field during and after a radiofrequency pulse.

Radiosurgery: Type of radiation therapy that focuses energy to a small area of a tumor, usually less than 3 to 4 centimeters in diameter. It does not involve surgery.

Randomized trial: Clinical trial involving at least two subgroups of patients comparing two or more different therapies, with the therapy selected by random assignment rather than by the patient or investigator.

Recreational therapist: Assists patients to engage in leisure activities such as cooking, arts and crafts, and music therapy that can provide a cognitive component to the "work" of physical rehabilitation.

Rehabilitation counselor: Assesses the goals of the patient and his or her return to work and family life.

Remission: Complete or partial disappearance of the signs and symptoms of disease in response to treatment; the period during which disease is under control.

Resectable: Able to be surgically removed.

Resection: Surgical removal of a tumor; *see also* Gross total resection and partial resection.

Sagittal image: An image that divides the brain into left and right hemispheres and is particularly good at showing tumors in the exact center of the brain.

Secondary malignancy: Cancer that develops as a result of previous cancer therapy.

Simulation: A practice treatment that allows the radiation team to determine exactly where the radiation treatment will be directed.

Speech therapist: Professionals who evaluate speech production, speech comprehension, and swallowing function.

Spinal tap: See *lumbar puncture*.

Status epilepticus: A condition in which the patient has repeated seizures or a seizure prolonged for at least 30 minutes.

Stereotactic radiosurgery (SRS): A radiation therapy technique using a large number of narrow, precisely aimed, highly focused beams of ionizing radiation. Beams aimed from many directions meet at a specific point. Usually only one treatment at high dose is planned.

Stereotactic biopsy: Removal of a small piece of the tumor using computer guidance, often with a thin needle placed through a tiny opening in the scalp and skull.

Stereotactic radiation: Type of radiation therapy that focuses energy to a small area of a tumor, usually less than 3 to 4 centimeters in diameter. It may be fractionated over several treatments.

Target volume: The three-dimensional portion of an organ or organs, identified from the patient's scans or x rays, to receive radiation therapy treatments.

Temporal lobe: Area in the cerebral hemispheres that contain both the auditory and visual pathways and the interpretation of sounds and spoken language for long-term memory.

Third ventricle: A spinal fluid-filled space in the center of the brain in communication with the lateral ventricles.

Thrombocytopenia: Low platelet count.

Whole brain radiation therapy: Radiation therapy delivered to the entire intracranial contents.

Index

Index

Motrin (ibuprophen), 155
Mouth sores, 173–174
MRI (magnetic resonance imaging), 9, 32,
      36, 37, 225
   follow-up, 39, 44, 44–45
   functional, 49–50
   guidance, 57–58
   intra-operative, 58
   post-surgery, 90
   principle of, 37–38
   procedure, 39
   and treatment planning, 82–83
MRS (magnetic resonance spectoscopy),
      48–49, 225
Multifocal tumors, 32, 33, 225
Multiple endocrine neoplasia type 1, 13t
Musella, Al, 128
Myelin, 4

N

National Cancer Institute (NCI), xviii, 128,
      211
National Comprehensive Cancer Network
      (NCCN), 86
National Institutes of Health (NIH), xix,
      128, 136, 211
   Center for Complementary and Alterna-
      tive Medicine, 135–136
Nausea, 21, 22, 152t
   treatment of, 99–101, 117, 173
NCCAM (National Center for Comple-
      mentary and Alternative Medi-
      cine), 135–136
Necrosis, radiation, 77, 83, 85
Negative margin, 226
Nerves, cranial, 8
Neulasta (Pegfilgrastim), 99
Neupogen (Filgrastim), 99
Neurofibromatosis, 13t
Neurological deficits, 21–22, 225
Neurological examination, 23–24, 225
Neuron, 4, 226
Neuronavigation, 58, 225
Neurontin (gabapentin), 157t
Neuropathologist, 26, 226
Neuropathy, 96–97
Neuropsychological evaluation, 195–196
Neuropsychologist, 68, 197–198
Neuropsychologists, 226
Neuroradiologist, 226
Neurosurgeon, 226
Neutropenia, 98–99, 148, 226

Neutrophils, 98, 226
New Approaches to Brain Tumor Therapy
      (NABTT), 128
Nocardia infection, 148
Nolvadex (tamoxifen), 113–114
Non-steroidal anti-inflammatory drugs
      (NSAIDS), 155, 165t
Noncancerous, definition, 226
Nondiagnostic biopsy, 54, 226
Nonlocalizing symptoms, 22, 226
Nortriptypine (Pamelor), 166
Nutrition, 12, 174, 176t

O

Occipital lobe, 6, 8, 226
Occupation, and incidence of tumor, 10–12,
      11t
Occupational therapy, 67, 68, 226
Odds ratio, 10, 11t
Off-label use, of medications, 115, 129,
      208, 226
Oligodendroglioma, 4, 33, 66–67, 226
Oligodentrocytes, 226
Ommaya reservoir, 107–109, 226
Oncologist, medical oncologist, 88–90, 151,
      225
Ondanseron (Zofran), 100
Open biopsy, 52, 60, 226
Organizations, list of, 213–215
orphan diseases, vii
Oxcarbazepine (Trileptal), 157t, 160t

P

Pain relievers, interaction with alcohol,
      167–168
Pallister-Hall syndrome, 13t
Pamelor (nortriptyline), 166
Pancreatitis, 157t
Paraplatin (carboplatin), 96, 164t
Parietal lobes, 6, 8, 226
Partial remission, 105–106, 226
Partial resection, 52–53, 55, 226–227
Partial seizure, 227
Pathologist, 25, 61–62
Pathology report, 25–26, 33, 227
Paxil (paroxetine), 166
PCV regimen, 86, 95, 167
Pegfilgrastim (Neulasta), 99
Penicillins, 165t
Personal appearance, changes in, 87–88
Personality, changes in, 21